TELOMERES AND EPIGENETICS
Modifying our genes

© Adolfo Pérez Agustí (2017-2024)

edicionesmasters@gmail.com

(Spain)

Nature gave us hunger and food, it gave us lungs and air, thirst and water. Nature instilled in us aggressiveness and taught us love, it became mysterious and gave us intelligence, it brought us diseases and provided us with remedies. Only the egomania of human beings has made them believe that behind the walls of a medical laboratory is the solution to their ills, that diseases can be avoided by inoculating poisons, and the health of one organ can be restored by damaging another. When, in a few years, humanity remembers how our generations were cured, with chemistry and invasive procedures that reach our insides, they will feel sorry for us.

Justification

From looking inside so much, we barely pay attention to the outside. But what is outside of us conditions us, pushes us and transforms us, more forcefully than what happens inside, since there is no determinism based on genetics, but only mutable characteristics.

Although cells carry out a series of complicated steps to translate their sequence of basic DNA blocks into proteins, through which they will carry out the vital functions of life, these changes will depend on genetic expression, almost always dependent on chronological, spatial changes. , or as a response to the environmental conditions in which the cell or individual is located. On the other hand, responses to the environment or developmental processes do not occur as a consequence of the activation of a single gene at a specific time, place or condition, but rather the coordinated expression of a set of them is usually necessary for the effect takes place. Therefore, everything that happens in the DNA chains is modifiable, even at will. The key lies in telomeres and epigenetics.

CHAPTER 1

There are no intelligence genes, although the interaction of thousands of them provides optimal results in the various branches of knowledge.

THE CELL

A cell is the basic unit of every organic being, the smallest element that can be considered alive and capable of acting autonomously.

All living organisms are made up of cells, and it is generally accepted that no organism is a living being if it does not consist of at least one cell.

The cell has an external or plasma membrane that surrounds it, rich in phospholipids, glycolipids and proteins, and its function is to maintain the cellular content by controlling what enters and leaves it. The entire internal content of the cell limited by the membrane is called *protoplasm*, and inside it are the nucleus and cytoplasm.

The human being is a multicellular organism equipped with *eukaryotic* cells that have genetic material in a single nucleus, which is surrounded by two lipid layers crossed by nuclear pores and linked to the *endoplasmic reticulum*. Inside the nucleus are DNA and RNA.

We have many billions of cells (an undetermined number) that have the extraordinary property of cooperating with each other to constitute very complex elements and ensure the survival of the organic whole.

For a better understanding, we will summarize some basic concepts:

Karyotype: Set of individual characteristics (number, size, appearance, shape, position of the centromere, etc.) of the chromosomes of a species that allows them to be identified as belonging to it.

Chromosomes: Structures found in the nucleus of cells that carry long fragments of DNA. They also contain proteins that help DNA exist in the proper form.

Each cell in the human body has 23 pairs of chromosomes, half come from the mother and half from the father. Two of the chromosomes, the X and the Y, determine the sex of the child. The father's chromosome determines sex.

Gene expression: The instructions provided by each gene to form a functional product, that is, a molecule necessary to perform a job in the cell. They can be expressed or silenced.

Phenotype: Interaction between genotype and epigenetics.

Genetics: Science that studies hereditary material at any level or dimension.

Gene: Chain of deoxyribonucleic acid (DNA) and molecular basis of inheritance, found in a fixed order on the chromosome. The human being has between 20 and 25,000 genes in each cell and they make up the human genome.

Genome: The total genetic material of an organism that includes genes as well as non-coding sequences.

Genomics: Study and application of the genome.

Genotype: Genetic information in the form of DNA of an organism.

Transgenesis: Process of transferring genes – information– from one organism to another.

DNA (deoxyribonucleic acid)

DNA, or deoxyribonucleic acid, is the hereditary material found in the nucleus of all cells in humans and other living organisms, more precisely referred to as nuclear DNA. However, a small part of DNA can also be found in the mitochondria (organelle in the cytoplasm that is responsible for cellular respiration and provides energy) and is called mitochondrial DNA or mtDNA. Both are electrical conductors and very sensitive to magnetic influences and ultraviolet radiation.

Basically, the main role of the DNA molecule is the long-term storage of information, which leads us to consider that the human being is basically an information organism, rather than an energy organism. The data or codes that will be used to give the necessary instructions that will build other components of the cells, such as proteins and RNA molecules, are stored there. These segments are more specifically referred to as *genes.* For this information to be used, it must be copied into other different units called RNA, which will be interpreted using the *genetic code*. The set of information is called the *genome*, while the DNA that constitutes it is the *genomic DNA*, and the set of all the information that corresponds to an organism is called the genotype, which, together with environmental factors, determines the characteristics of the organism. that is, its *phenotype*.

DNA molecules specify the sequence by which the 20 amino acids in the human body form the thirty thousand necessary proteins.

DNA is a polymer of nucleotides, a compound made up of many simple units connected together. Each *nucleotide* is made up of a sugar or pentose (deoxyribose), a nitrogenous base and a phosphate group that acts as a linker to the structure. The union of the nitrogenous base (cytosine, adenine, guanine and thymine) with the *pentose* (deoxyribose) forms a *nucleoside*; this, joining with phosphoric acid, gives us a nucleotide, while the union of the nucleotides together gives us a polynucleotide, in this case deoxyribonucleic acid.

These nucleotides are arranged in two long chains that form a spiral in the shape of a double helix and which is perceived as a spiral staircase, where the base pairs form the rungs of the ladder and the sugar and phosphate molecules form the sides of the ladder stairs.

In living organisms, DNA occurs as a double chain of nucleotides, in which the two strands are linked to each other by connections called hydrogen bonds that act as a source of attraction between two atoms. The genetic information is deposited there thanks to the sequential arrangement of the four nitrogenous bases along the chain. Their composition of nucleic acids, Adenine (A) and Guanine (G), and pyrimidines such as Cytosine (C) and Thymine (T), allows them to be complementary to each other: A pairs with T, and C with G. This pairing is maintained due to the action of hydrogen bonds between both bases, forming base pairs that give rise to the rungs of the ladder directed towards the center and perpendicular to the axis of the molecule, while the sugar and phosphate molecules They form the sides of the staircase.

DNA in humans contains around 3 billion bases and these are 99% similar in people. These bases are sequenced differently to carry out the different information that needs to be transmitted. Another property is that they can make copies of themselves. Thus, each new DNA has a copy of the old DNA from which the copy is made.

It can also shape metallic structures in the same way it shapes protein synthesis.

Mitochondrial DNA

Each cell contains hundreds of thousands of mitochondria in the cytoplasm that house small amounts of DNA known as *mitochondrial* DNA or mtDNA, which contains 37 genes. Thirteen of these genes provide instructions for making enzymes involved in energy production through oxidative phosphorylation, and it is estimated that up to 90% of cellular energy in the form of ATP is produced in this way. The rest of the genes help in making *transfer RNA* (tRNA) and *ribosomal RNA* (rRNA) molecules that cause protein synthesis.

Replication

DNA replication, which occurs only once in each cell generation, requires many enzymes and a large amount of energy in the form of ATP (adenosine triphosphate). The initiation of replication, or *G1 phase*, always occurs in a certain group of nucleotides, which requires, among others, *helicase* enzymes to break hydrogen bonds and *topoisomerases* to relieve tension, and single-strand binding proteins to maintain separate the open chains. This phase lasts between 6 and 12 hours, and during this time the cell doubles its size and mass due to the continuous synthesis of all its components.

Afterwards, the cells go into a *G2 phase* in order, among other things, to recover energy for the next phase of cell division, which lasts between 3 and 4 hours. This process provides a nucleus with twice as many nuclear proteins and allows each chromosome to duplicate and form two identical *chromatids*.

DNA replication in humans occurs at a speed of 50 nucleotides per second, but these nucleotides have to be assembled and available in the nucleus along with the energy to join them.

Once the molecule is opened, an area known as the replication bubble forms where the *replication forks* are located, the juncture when the DNA is self-replicating. Through the action of *DNA polymerase*, the new nucleotides enter the hairpin and link with the corresponding nucleotide of the original strand (A with T, C with G).

One chain will form a continuous copy, while the other will form a series of short fragments known as *Okazaki fragments*. The chain that is synthesized continuously is known as the leading chain and the one that is synthesized in fragments is known as the lagging chain.

For DNA polymerase to work, the presence, at the beginning of each new fragment, of small RNA units known as primers is necessary, which will allow other enzymes to be activated and remove the RNA fragments and place the DNA nucleotides in their place. . Finally, a *DNA ligase* will join them to the growing chain.

RNA

Ribonucleic Acid (RNA) or Adenosine Ribonucleic Acid, was discovered after DNA and was not restricted to the nucleus of eukaryotes, since it is also found in the cytoplasm and ribosomes. Let us remember that ribosomes are 2/3 RNA, a type called *ribosomal RNA* (rRNA), and 1/3 proteins. A typical cell contains 10 times more RNA than DNA.

It is an important molecule with long chains of nucleotides (a nucleotide contains a nitrogenous base, a ribose sugar, and a phosphate) and like DNA, RNA is of vital importance for living beings, containing adenine bases, cytosine, guanine and uracil (instead of thymine).

While DNA is defined as a nucleic acid that contains the genetic instructions used in the development and function of all known living organisms, RNA molecules are involved in protein synthesis and, often, in the transmission of information. genetics. Unlike DNA, RNA comes in a variety of forms and types. Thus, while DNA is seen as a double helix and a spiral staircase, RNA can be more than one type, usually single-stranded, while DNA is generally double-stranded. On the other hand, the RNA chain is shorter and its appearance is like a band, not a double helix.

The deoxyribose sugar in DNA is less reactive because of CH bonds and is stable under alkaline conditions.

It has small grooves where the damaging enzyme can bind, making it more difficult for the enzyme to attack the DNA. RNA, on the other hand, is not stable in alkaline conditions and has large grooves, which makes it easier to be attacked by enzymes, although it is more resistant to damage by ultraviolet rays.

To duplicate itself, DNA needs another molecule to act as a messenger or collaborator that copies the information, and that molecule is RNA, whose fundamental function is to transcribe DNA orders and thus form new proteins, transferring the genetic code from the nucleus. to the ribosome.

This process prevents DNA from having to leave the nucleus, keeping it, along with the genetic code, protected from damage. Without RNA, protein synthesis could never occur.

RNA is formed from DNA through a process called transcription, which involves using enzymes such as polymerases. There is a type of RNA called messenger RNA (mRNA) that transports information from DNA to structures called ribosomes. These ribosomes are made of proteins and ribosomal RNA (rRNA). All of them join together and form a complex that can read messenger RNAs and translate the information that they lead to the formation of proteins. This requires the help of transfer RNA or tRNA.

Information flows (with the exception of reverse transcription) from DNA to RNA using DNA as a template, and then to the protein through the translation process (construction of an amino acid sequence - polypeptide - with the information provided by the molecule). RNA).

All 20 amino acids are represented in the genetic code. Methionine (actually formyl-methionine, f-Met) is always the first amino acid of the polypeptide chain, and is often removed at the end of the process.

Some RNAs are enzymes and although it was previously believed that only proteins could be enzymes, it is now known that they can adopt complex tertiary structures and act as biological catalysts. RNA enzymes are known as ribozymes, and they exhibit many of the characteristics of a classical enzyme, such as an active site, a binding site for a substrate, and a binding site for a cofactor, such as a metal ion. One of the first ribozymes to be discovered was RNase P, a ribonuclease that is involved in the generation of RNA molecules.

Specific:

Messenger Ribonucleic Acid (mRNA) is the template for the construction of the protein.

Ribosomal Ribonucleic Acid (rRNA) is found in the site where the protein is built: the ribosome, the organelles of the cell where proteins are synthesized.

Transfer Ribonucleic Acid (tRNA) is the transporter that places the appropriate amino acid in the corresponding site.

RNA has the *sugar ribose* instead of deoxyribose and the base uracil (U) replaces thymine (T).

RNA has a single strand, although tRNA can form a cloverleaf-shaped structure due to the complementarity of its base pairs.

The mRNA, regardless of the organism from which it comes, can initiate protein synthesis.

Cellular division

In humans, when we talk about mitosis we are referring to the nucleus. During mitosis the replicated chromosomes are positioned near the middle of the cell and then segregate in such a way that each resulting cell receives one copy of each original chromosome.

In cell division we can distinguish several phases that are difficult to separate, since it is a dynamic process.

Interphase is not part of mitosis and in it the DNA has been replicated, but the condensed structure of the chromosome has not been formed. The nuclear membrane is still intact to protect the DNA molecules from mutation. It covers phases G1 (growth and maturation), S (copying DNA),

G2 (preparation for division), and if that cell is no longer going to divide anymore, it enters what is called the G0 period. If, on the other hand, that cell is going to divide again, it enters the G1 period again.

Prophase, where the chromatin becomes visible, the nucleolus disappears, the centrioles move and the mitotic spindle forms, forming chromosomes. Lasts 35 to 40 minutes.

Prometaphase, with the cell membrane dissolved and the chromosomes beginning to move.

Metaphase, with the spindle fibers aligning the chromosomes in the middle of the nucleus, prevents premature progression to the next phase.

Anaphase, where the pairs of chromosomes move to opposite sides of the cell and two copies are formed with the original genetic information. This phase is very quick, lasting only three or four minutes.

Telophase, with chromosomes dispersed and new membranes, chromatin and nucleolus forming. There are already two identical cells with their nuclei.

Cynothesis, where the daughter cells are already separated and have a nucleus, as well as a complete copy of the genome of the original cell.

Apoptosis is cell death by fragmentation, but it is a normal process that benefits the organism as a whole. It occurs after several divisions and its remains are reused by macrophages.

Meiosis is a type of sexual reproduction. It is a special type of cell division necessary for sexual reproduction in eukaryotes.

Reviewing the genes

Genes are segments of DNA that are coded to form a specific protein. These proteins are responsible for the expression of the *phenotype*, the external manifestation of a set of hereditary characteristics that depend on both genes and the environment. *Polygenic inheritance* is the set responsible for many characters such as weight, shape, height, color and metabolism that are governed by the cumulative effect of many genes. Height in humans is a type of polygenic inheritance.

Chromosomal abnormalities include inversion, insertion, duplication, and loss of a DNA fragment from a chromosome. Since DNA is information, and it has a starting point, an inversion produces an inactive or altered protein. Likewise, a duplication can alter the gene product.

A gene is nothing more than a fragment of DNA, that is, a set of nucleotides linked together, with information for a given character, in such a way that a chromosome can be considered as a set of genes.

Genes determine the hereditary characteristics of each cell or organism, the hereditary material found within the nucleus of the cell. It is estimated that humans have genes that cause aging, but this is a hypothesis.

Each person has two copies of each gene, one inherited from each parent. These are mostly similar in all people, but a small number of genes (less than 1 percent of the total) are slightly different between people, determining paternity.

A gene can contain several thousand codons, each coding for an amino acid. A codon is a triplet of nucleotides, the basic unit of information in the translation process. This correspondence is the basis of the genetic code that allows the mRNA sequence to be translated into the amino acid sequence that constitutes the protein. There are 64 different codons per combination of the 4 nucleotides in each of the 3 positions of the triplet, but only 61 code for amino acids. Except for methionine and tryptophan, which are coded by a single codon, amino acids can be coded by 2, 3, 4 or 6 different codons. Codons that code for the same amino acid often have the first two nucleotides the same, only changing the third.

Chromosomal abnormalities

Diseases of this type must be considered as failed evolutionary attempts, since the human karyotype is in continuous evolution.

In a chromosome there may be altered regions or loci and even mutations or chromosomopathies, alterations in the number of genes or in their order within the chromosomes that are due to errors during gametogenesis or in the first divisions of the zygote.

Chromosomal abnormalities occur in 0.48% of live human births. They also account for 25-30% of spontaneous abortions.

Trisomy 21, or Down syndrome, occurs globally in 1 in every 700 births. This anomaly is not transmitted genetically, but is acquired. This disorder occurs when a person has 47 chromosomes instead of the usual 46. Most cases occur when there is an extra copy of chromosome 21.

As a percentage, in women up to 20 years old, trisomy 21 occurs in 1 every 2,000 births. In women up to 30 years old, in 1 every thousand births. From the age of 35 it is 1 in 350, and at 45 it is one in 30.

Other trisomies, such as 13 and 18, do not survive.

Mitochondrial diseases are transmitted maternally. We know that mitochondria contain DNA smaller than nuclear DNA and that they are found in the cytoplasm. Those affected by *NARD syndrome*, which is caused by mutations in mitochondrial DNA, suffer from proximal muscle weakness with sensory neuropathy, ataxia, and retinitis pigmentosa.

Those affected by *Leigh syndrome,* a progressive degenerative brain disease, suffer from lesions of the brain stem and basal ganglia. Its prevalence at birth has been estimated at 1/36,000. The onset of symptoms typically occurs before 12 months of age but, in rare cases, can occur during adolescence, or even early adulthood.

Myoclonic epilepsy is usually associated with an alteration located on chromosome 6. It is common to have episodes of strong jerks of the upper limbs and to a lesser extent the lower limbs, which usually appear preferentially after waking up or associated with deprivation of dream.

In *genetic mental deficiency* or oligophrenia, there are abnormal reactions to a stimulus, with problems in learning, instincts and consciousness. It may be due to trauma at the time of birth, or brain conditions. Also to polygenic systems (multifactorial inheritance) or to some anomalies in the sexual chromosome constitution.

Chronic *myeloid leukemia* is a type of cancer that begins in certain blood producing cells of the bone marrow, caused by the formation of an abnormal gene called BCR-ABL.

Patients with *Hutchinson-Gilford progeria* have an autosomal dominant mutation on chromosome 1q, producing a toxic protein called progerin.

Is there biological determinism?

Biological determinism tells us about the belief that human development and even behavior are controlled by an individual's genes. According to this inconsistent theory, both the shared norms of behavior and the social and physiological differences that exist between groups, basically differentiated by race, place or sex, derive from inherited characteristics.

Particularities, therefore, would be immutable, as much as genetic diseases, another fatalistic error that has led millions of people to resignation.

Genetic determinism tries to differentiate individuals based on their genetic structure, but it too often forgets that we are body, mind and spirit, and that every biological process is susceptible to change if certain circumstances occur or we know how. Therefore, we must consider genetics as a rapid adaptation mechanism, but not immutable and, of course, improvable. What's more, evolution is proof of how species have adapted with respect to their ancestors and have made a leap in the evolutionary assessment scale. If everything were determined by genetic characteristics, the human being would be a clone of our ancestors.

So, once we have clarified that *strict biological determinism* does not exist, both in biology and in psychological characteristics, we see that the phenotype is the expression of the genotype depending on a certain environment, in principle, the visible manifestation of the genotype. , although this explanation falls very short. Therefore, we can study the genotype by observing the DNA, while the phenotype requires the observation of its morphology, development, biochemical properties, physiology and behavior, all influenced by the environment.

In conclusion, once the human egg has been fertilized by a human sperm, there is only one determinism: there will be a human being.

CHAPTER 2

THEORIES OF AGING

Why do we age? Although the question has been raised for hundreds of years, the mysteries that control human life have not yet been discovered.

Over the last few decades, many theories have been proposed to explain the aging process, but none of them seem to be fully satisfactory. Instead, we see that these theories interact with each other and a mixture of elements contributes to aging.

In this book, however, we will only discuss the three main theories of aging: cellular senescence, epigenetics, and telomere shortening.

Cellular senescence

Recent studies suggest that cellular senescence could be a cellular model of organismal aging. Accumulations of senescent cells were found in vivo in mammals with increasing age, and at sites of age-related pathologies.

Cellular senescence is an apparent state of irreversible growth arrest, which was first introduced by Hayflick and Moorhead in 1961. They found that normal human fibroblasts cultured in vitro had limited replicative potential and stopped growing - they had lost the ability to divide-, and that despite having ample space and nutrients in the growing medium.

Based on this, two general models have been proposed to explain how cellular senescence can contribute to aging. First, senescent cells in tissues can accumulate to the point where the strength and functional capacity of the tissues are compromised. A second model proposes that senescence in stem cells limits their regenerative potential which eventually leads to a progressive loss of tissue strength and functional capacity. As we will later see, cellular senescence can be triggered by a series of mechanisms, such as telomere shortening and DNA damage. Because cells are the fundamental building blocks of our body, it is logical to assume that cellular changes contribute to the aging process.

The Hayflick Limit

In 1961, and in contradiction to what was thought at the time, Leonard Hayflick and Paul Moorhead discovered that human cells derived from embryonic tissues could only divide a finite number of times. They observed that, in laboratory cultures, cells stopped dividing after an average of 50 cumulative doublings, but could increase or decrease under certain conditions. This phenomenon of growth arrest after a period of apparently normal cell proliferation is known as the Hayflick limit, or replicative senescence (RS).

Both worked with fibroblasts, a cell type found in connective tissue widely used in research, although SR has been found in other types of cells: keratinocytes, endothelial cells, lymphocytes, adrenocortical cells, vascular smooth muscle cells, chondrocytes, etc. It is also observed in cells derived from embryonic tissues, in cells from adults of all ages and in cells taken from many animals: mice, chickens, Galapagos tortoises, etc. The research was reviewed by Hayflick in 1994.

Early results suggested that CPD (cancer of unknown primary origin) cells could last longer under certain conditions and the longevity of a species could derive from very specific cells. For example, the cells of the Galapagos tortoises, which can live more than a century and their cells divide about 110 times, had different characteristics from those of the mouse, which divide approximately 15 times, much less than in humans.

Furthermore, cells taken from patients with Werner syndrome (WS) - accelerated aging due to trisomy of chromosome 8 - have much less CPD than normal cells. There are exceptions and certain cell lines can divide indefinitely without reaching RS. They are said to be immortal and include embryonic germ cells and most tumor-derived cell lines, such as HeLa cells, the immortal human cancer cells. Some types of rat cells have also been claimed to be able to evade SR, and more recently some mouse cells have been found to be immortal under certain culture conditions.

Biomarkers of Cellular Senescence

The discovery of RS sparked considerable interest and the phenotype of cellular senescence in human fibroblasts has been characterized by a number of features, termed Adda di Fagagna biomarkers. The most obvious biomarker is growth arrest, that is, cells stop dividing, which can be detected by different methods. Even vigorously dividing cultures are heterogeneous and contain a percentage of growth-arrested cells. This percentage increases progressively until all the cells in the population are at rest, that is, they have stopped dividing. Growth arrest in RS appears irreversible, in the sense that growth factors cannot stimulate the division of all cells, although senescent cells can remain metabolically active for long periods of time.

Another important biomarker is cell morphology. Although cells mature in vitro, they undergo progressive morphological changes. In fact, a senescent confluent culture has a smaller cell density than a young confluent culture, although this also occurs because senescent cells are more sensitive to inhibition of cell-cell contact.

Lysosomes, organelles that break down cellular waste, increase in number and size in senescent cells.

The expression levels of several genes change during cellular aging in vitro. An important type of gene overexpressed in senescent cells are inflammatory regulators such as interleukin 6 (IL6).

Some studies support a role for proinflammatory proteins secreted by senescent cells in driving senescence, which may lead to positive feedback loops and the induction of senescence in normal cells near senescent cells.

Epigenetics and DNA damage

Studies showed that cellular senescence is commonly triggered by various forms of DNA damage. Mutant mice that are deficient in DNA repair show premature senescence and progeroid phenotypes, suggesting the involvement of DNA damage-induced senescence in aging. Sources of DNA damage include external sources, such as tobacco smoke, ionizing radiation, electromagnetic pollution, and genotoxic drugs, as well as cell-intrinsic sources, such as replication errors, programmed double-strand breaks, and DNA damaging agents.

Reactive oxygen species (ROS), such as superoxide anion, hydroxyl radical, hydrogen peroxide, and nitric oxide, are normal byproducts of metabolism that were produced in the mitochondria, and are believed to be a major source of damage in the DNA.

ROS can damage mitochondrial DNA (mtDNA) and proteins, and mutant mtDNA in turn are more likely to produce ROS byproducts. Therefore, a positive feedback loop of ROS is established. With age, the number of mtDNA mutants increases and mitochondrial functions decrease, leading to an increase in ROS production.

Increased generation of ROS can cause lipid peroxidation, protein damage, and various types of DNA lesions in cells. Therefore, they are considered important factors in the mechanisms of diseases such as diabetes, cancer, atherosclerosis, heart attacks, Alzheimer's disease, as well as aging. Evidence has shown that species that live longer generally show greater resistance to cellular oxidative stress and lower levels of mitochondrial ROS production, compared to species that live shorter.

Telomere shortening

Telomeres lose a little of their length during each cell division. Since replicative DNA polymerases are not capable of replicating telomeres, and telomerase (which could replicate telomeres) is not always expressed in normal mammalian somatic cells, telomeres become too short to replicate after a fixed number of cell divisions. .

Telomeres are particularly susceptible to the accumulation of DNA damage with age, and this damage to telomeres is not always repaired because of shelterin or telosome, a protein complex that regulates the activity of telomerase and prevents the access of proteins. of DNA repair to telomeres. Therefore, DNA damage at telomeres is persistent, although reversible, inducing cellular senescence.

Calorie restriction

Some studies have shown that calorie restriction (i.e., a 20-40% reduction in caloric intake) extends lifespan in several species ranging from yeast to rodents.

One possible explanation is that caloric restriction reduced the production of reactive oxygen species by mitochondria. Additionally, calorie restriction induces autophagy which removes harmful proteins and organelles, thereby reducing cumulative damage to the cell. However, this phenomenon is still not conclusive in humans, but research seems to confirm the effectiveness of a low-calorie diet, especially in the hours preceding sleep.

Evolutionary aging

The aging of cells seems like the inevitable wear and tear of everything around us. Cars rust, tires wear out, cars head to the junkyard. Over time, things inevitably head toward disorder. Is it, after all, a law of physics? The second law of thermodynamics? ("while all mechanical work can be transformed into heat, not all heat can be transformed into mechanical work") Some scientists therefore concluded that the mere conception of stopping or reversing the aging of cells was therefore absurd. Poor scientists who, locked in their laboratory, forget the complexity of the human being: body, mind and spirit. In fact, the evolution of human beings has been surprising and each new adaptation makes them stronger and longer lived.

For centuries, life has slowly evolved into more and more complexity. If the species itself is perpetuated through the immortal lineage of germ cells, then why can't we live many more years? Remarkably, cells think, adapt, and seek to essentially survive and perpetuate themselves. The cells that made us could be traced and allow us to connect with our ancestors from thousands of years ago, even with those who lived many millions of years ago in a more elemental form, in the form of bacteria. Still, the collection of cells that make up the body are destined to live a few decades. Or not? Our cells adapt well, but they have not yet found a way to stay much longer.

Immortal cells

Therefore, the first clue on the path to understanding cellular aging is that some cells seem to escape aging in the process of perpetuating the species. And this probably does not depend on the process of sexual reproduction (production of eggs and sperm), since some advanced animals can perpetuate themselves without sex in a process known as parthenogenesis (virgin birth) with only female egg cells involved.

The second clue is that some mortal somatic cells seem to find their way to immortality in vitro, when they only breathe, eat and rest. In work on cellular aging, George Gey of Johns Hopkins University reported that cells from a patient with cervical cancer proliferated abundantly in the laboratory. Over the years, it became clear that these and many other cancer cells did not necessarily age like the normal cells studied by Hayflick. These first cultured cancer cells isolated by Gey were designated "HeLa" after Henrietta Lacks.

In addition to the immortality of cancer-derived cells, it became evident that normal cells could be transformed into cancer cells in the laboratory using certain tumor viruses such as papillomavirus and a related virus called SV40.

In 1965, Hilary Koprowski's group showed that the SV40 virus could first extend the cellular lifespan of normal human cells in the laboratory and then, more rarely, immortalize them. What a paradox. The same cell that kills a human being can make him immortal. One of the strangest things was that the virus was somehow able to extend the lifespan of the cells, but they still suffered a type of aging called a "crisis." And in the cells that had gone into crisis there was almost always the presence of chromosomes fused at the ends (the telomeres). Thus, telomeric fusions accompanied this crisis event. The correct path was indicated.

Another clue was that around one in 10 million cells in the crisis phase in the presence of the SV40 virus could find their way to immortality. It seems little, but the exception is always the clue to the great discovery. Mathematics can make us wrong and we must look for the conclusions of quantum indeterminism.

Therefore, there are clues that the mechanisms of cellular aging and immortalization may not be as complex as one might think. But what are these mechanisms?

Some of the earliest research on cellular aging suggests that there must be some kind of molecular mechanism. When Len's cells were thawed, even after many years, they began to proliferate again in the dish, and despite the passage of chronological time, they had not aged, but continued right where they left off and proliferated with the same number of doublings. as if they had never been frozen. Time, so important to us, was not a determining factor in aging.

To rule out unfrozen chronological time as a cause, Robert Dell'Orco at the Noble Foundation in Oklahoma showed that cells kept unfrozen, for long periods of time, still proliferated the same number of duplications as those that had not been especially treated. Thus, Dell'Orco concluded that aging human cells were not measuring metabolic time, but rather were "counting" cell divisions.

Since, we believe, they have no brain or any known memory mechanism that could count and remember how many times they had divided, they followed what their nature dictated.

A couple of years later, Woody Wright performed a difficult test to see where the supposed clock was inside the cell and he did so by swapping the nuclei of young and old cells. Of course, it is within the central nucleus of the cell, the master blueprint of life called resident DNA. The experiments showed that the nucleus of an old cell drifted towards a young cell, and vice versa. So these experiments indicated that the cellular aging clock counted only cell divisions and those located in the nucleus.

The DNA molecule has regions, the genes, which are the instructions to perform functions such as the proteins that function within the cell.

But there are other regions in DNA that have, for example, long stretches of DNA with repeating sequences that are not technically genes.

It is possible that there may be progressive changes in these non-coding regions of DNA that, since they did not code for proteins, instead function like a clock.

The molecules that attach to the DNA strand to "photocopy" each time a cell repeats cannot copy the ends, specifically the telomeres. The result would be that the cell would be fine for some period of time, but the progressive shortening of the ends of the chromosome over time would eventually cause the cell to have severe damage leading to cellular aging. But then how do we explain the immortality of the germ line and cancer cells? In the case of the immortal germline, Olovnikov proposed that there existed a special type of DNA copying machinery that had not yet been discovered, which could reproduce the same ends. In these cells, DNA could be faithfully reproduced each time a cell divides, allowing the cells to potentially live forever.

Cellular renewal

Bone cells: every 10 years

Heart: slowly, 1% a year

Red blood cells: every 120 days

Bone marrow: continuously

Stomach: every two weeks

Skin: every month

Brain: never

Intestine: every five days

Liver: every 100 days

The cells that renew most easily are: hair, nails, skin, oral mucosa, digestive system, blood, muscles, bones, liver.

Loss of telomeres in cellular aging

From a mess (including telomere-less chromosome pairs that fuse together to try to heal broken ones), the telomerase gene is rarely activated, resulting in stabilization of telomeres at a relatively short length.

Cells begin life with a TRF (terminal restriction fragment) length of approximately 15 thousand base pairs (kbp) of DNA and shorten to an average length of approximately 5 kbp at the Hayflick limit. Viruses like SV40 can extend cell lifespan to an even shorter length and then arrest cells in crisis. The telomere changes with age.

Clearly, the loss of telomeric DNA may offer a mechanism to understand why cells eventually stop dividing. It is as if the broken DNA strand puts a brake on the cell's ability to proliferate. These brakes, in turn, are likely to be overcome by tumor viruses.

Although some critics doubted the causal connection of telomere shortening and telomerase in cellular aging and immortalization, sheer imaging evidence reinforced the thesis.

During mitosis, the two centromeres are separated by the spindle, and as a result of the mechanical stress, a new fragmentation is generated, and the two resulting chromosomes do not have functional telomeres, thus leading to a new fusion cycle. A variety of aberrant chromosomes are produced by this mechanism. However, as long as telomerase is not activated, the newly formed chromosome will remain without a functional telomere, and cells subject to these cycles eventually die. However, if cells have a shortened telomere and active telomerase, this can actively produce aberrant and stable chromosomes. Under these conditions, the opportunity to form a modified chromosome will be significantly increased.

Telomerase and cancer

Studies using cell culture models indicated that to become immortal, cells need to overcome two critical stages, Mortality stages 1 (M1) and 2 (M2). These observations of immortalized cells in vitro led to the proposal that cancer cells activate telomerase to grow immortally.

Are cancer cells immortal, then, due to an activation of telomerase? In 1989, Gregg Morin of the University of California at Davis succeeded in measuring telomeres by telomerase activity, concluding that they were immortal through a process called HeLa, the study with laboratory cells. While telomerase did not achieve this effect in normal mortal cells, the definitive answer about the possible association of cancer and telomerase awaited a new and sensitive means of detecting the activity of the molecule. It was puzzling, until a new, more sensitive technique called "TRAP" made it possible for the first time to reach a conclusion.

A large-scale study of many types of cancer showed that immortal cancer cell lines were positive for telomerase activity, while none of the 22 normal cells showed the presence of telomerase. Interestingly, the telomeres of the tumor cells also showed activity, while the normal tissues showed no changes. This not only supported the association of telomerase with immortality, always speaking of tumor cells, it also suggested that telomerase could be a target for diagnosis and therapy. However, the puzzle of how telomerase was activated or deactivated remained.

The remaining question was, could we actually find the genes for telomerase components and finally test the telomere hypothesis in cellular aging and immortalization? If cancer cells could be immortal, why couldn't they be normal ones? Dr. Carol Greider demonstrated that telomeric repeats in an aquatic organism called Tetrahymena were made by an enzyme that provided the information to make the correct order of DNA. For this pioneering work on telomerase, Elizabeth Blackburn, and Jack Szostack won a Nobel Prize.

That naturally immortal single-celled animal, the Tetrahymena, reflected the ancient immortal origins of life as described by August Weismann. But was this enzyme actually the key to aging and immortalization? We remind you that telomerase is a combination of protein and RNA. The RNA binds to the telomere and encodes the correct synthesis of 'TTAGGG' at the telomeric end thus extending its length.

In 1995 it was specified that by removing RNA, laboratory HeLa cells could be forced to return from their immortal state to a mortal one and stop dividing after 23-26 doublings.

The telomerase gene would simply have to be transferred into mortal cells. They then grow normal cells to old age with and without the added gene. Of course, the DNA containing the gene had to be manipulated so that the gene could not be turned off when it was in the cell. If adding the gene extended the life of the cell or even created immortalized human cells, the experiment would be a success.

At the end, the cells with the added telomerase gene lived longer and longer. In fact, they showed no evidence of aging. One gene was enough to stop the aging of human cells. For some reason, that gene (the catalytic component of telomerase) was turned off in somatic cells, leading to telomere shortening when the cells divided, while remaining intact in germline cells. The next question was whether we could use the gene to test the role of cellular aging in human aging.

The evolution of aging

There has been much speculation about why we evolved as a deadly species. A simple answer, but difficult to assume and possibly wrong, is that human beings must die, as well as live. The problem is that people are now living much longer than before, and we are seeing an increase in age-related degenerative diseases, linked to the aging of cells in tissues throughout the body.

So is it possible to reverse the biological markers of aging by activating telomerase? It's that easy? Can we, then, reverse or prevent age-related degenerative disease? My best guess is that older individuals at risk of serious illness could try herbal extracts, for example, astragalus root, but it seems that our scientists do not show much interest, perhaps because medicinal plants are not patentable.

In the case of life-threatening age-related diseases, is there a more powerful method to restore cell life to the body for therapeutic purposes? One method to achieve this could be gene therapy.

As was done in the first laboratory tests of telomerase, we could put the gene into a virus and use it to spread the gene throughout the body, adding the gene to cells and potentially resetting the telomere clock.

Stress-induced premature senescence

A number of factors can accelerate and/or trigger cellular senescence, one of which is oxidative stress. Typically, cell culture conditions include 20% oxygen and these were the conditions initially used by Hayflick and Moorhead and most subsequent studies. The way in which toxic stress (let's not forget that there is healthy stress) can accelerate the appearance of the senescent phenotype in cells has been considered as another form of cellular senescence called stress-induced premature senescence.

It is not surprising that, depending on the dose of stress endured, a cell population reacts in different ways. For example, a high cytotoxic dose will cause such an amount of damage that cellular biochemical activities will decrease, leading to cell death by necrosis. The level of damage suffered by cells determines whether programmed cell death -apoptosis- can occur or, if the damage is minor, senescence. Since a cell population is not homogeneous, the dosage of the stress factor will shift the percentage of cells that execute each of the possible programs depending on the amount of stress, that is: adaptive stress, oxidative stress, cellular stress, senescence, apoptosis and necrosis.

In addition to O_2, other sources of oxidative damage, such as H_2O_2 and stress factors -for example ethanol and ionizing radiation- can induce SIPS (points indicative of stress) in many types of proliferative cells, such as lung and skin fibroblasts. , endothelial cells, melanocytes and retinal pigment epithelial cells. The list of stressors that can cause SIPS is constantly growing and instead of chronic stress, SIPS can be induced based on one or several short exposures to stressors. Oncogenes can also induce senescence, since because organisms and cells are constantly exposed to stress factors, senescent cells in vivo can arise not only from cell divisions, but from cells exposed to stress.

With all this, the connection between the aging of organisms and cellular senescence remains a topic of controversy, despite decades of study.

Except in the postpartum period, there is no relationship between the number of CPDs (cancer-producing cells) that the cells can support and the age of the donor. A study conducted on centenarians found no difference in what CPDs taken from centenarians could support compared to cells from young donors. As we know, cells at birth from patients with certain progeroid syndromes have fewer divisions than cells from healthy controls. This, however, could be the result of increased cell death or cell cycle exit for reasons unrelated to RS. In fact, senescent cells from Werner syndrome patients have different gene expression patterns and biomarkers of senescence. It should also be noted that people, even the very old, never run out of proliferating cells.

Furthermore, because of the positive correlation between body size and longevity, perhaps cells taken from long-lived animals support more CPDs due to differences in size, not due to differences in longevity. Senescent cells and biomarkers associated with senescence can be found in various human tissues in vivo associated with both aging and pathology.

Interestingly, stress-prone tissues seem to be the most affected. For example, fibroblasts cultured in the distal lower extremities of patients with venous reflux, which precede the development of venous ulcers, show characteristics of senescent cells. Similar results also relate cellular senescence to atherosclerosis. In mouse liver, one study estimated that more than 20% of hepatocytes were potentially senescent. Senescent cells have also been found in other mouse tissues, although possibly through telomere-independent mechanisms.

Because senescent cells can secrete proinflammatory cytokines and other factors that alter the tissue microenvironment, they may contribute to altered cellular and tissue function. Even a small percentage of senescent cells, in fact, can interfere with tissue homeostasis and function. In fact, there is evidence that senescent cells contribute to age-related pathologies such as osteoarthritis and skin aging. Senescent cells could also contribute to increased inflammatory levels, creating a positive feedback loop.

One study reported that clearance of senescent cells delays aging-associated disorders and we have found that there are senescent cells in vivo without telomere shortening. One hypothesis is that senescent cells in vivo are not caused by telomere shortening, but by various stress factors.

Some data indicate that chronic stressors may accelerate the risk of a number of age-related diseases by prematurely aging the immune response.

There also appears to be a relationship between stress resistance and aging, and extended longevity as greater stress resistance. Cells from older individuals who are more susceptible to stress exhibit higher levels of biomarkers of senescence in general.

There is no doubt that there are changes that occur with age at the cellular level. Some genetic interventions that regulate aging appear to influence tissue homeostasis by affecting senescence, cell proliferation, and cell death.

Evolution does not favor long life, although it does favor strength and optimizes development mechanisms for reproduction. Once an organism has passed its genes to the next generation, perhaps evolution stops and the same genes responsible for the growth and maturation of that organism will end up inadvertently killing it.

Therefore, perhaps some hormones such as GH and genes involved in insulin-like signaling regulate growth and development early in life, and later contribute to aging.

Neuroendocrine mechanisms that control development can extend after maturation and give rise to a regulatory cascade that results in age-related changes. Excessive nutrition can accelerate maturation (stronger children), but decrease life expectancy. Therefore, perhaps we should view aging as a developmental consequence linked to the impact of the endocrine system on aging.

In some tissues, such as the immune system, decreased proliferative capacity may play a role in age-related degeneration. Successive spleen and bone marrow transplants gave inconclusive results, but it appears that a slight decrease in proliferative capacity occurs in vivo even though the cells had to divide much more than 50 times.

Cardiomyocyte turnover in humans decreases with age. Therefore, there are aging mechanisms intrinsic to cells. These may be related to the senescent phenotype, but undoubtedly to other processes as well. Cells from older donors were initially reported to have a slower proliferative capacity. This effect, known as the latent period, occurs because fewer cells are in the replication cycle, not because they need more time to divide. Instead, alterations in gene expression, resulting from quality control defects, allow errors to accumulate as cells divide, leading to cells with diminished function.

CHAPTER 3

HUMAN LONGEVITY

It does not seem that we live in a wonderful time, medically speaking, because despite the fact that there are more hospitals than ever (a clear sign that the health of the population is bad, very bad), half of the population of the United States has problems with Chronic diseases and life expectancy appear to be in decline, and for most, the idea of living to 100 years of age might seem like a pipe dream, or a punishment. Imagine if we talk to you about 120 years of life, the ideal achievable according to the latest discoveries.

Oldest cities

Older people are increasing in Spain and on January 1, 2014, the National Institute of Statistics (INE) registered 88,821 people over 95, compared to 83,452 in 2013. In July 2016, a total of 17,423 people had overcome the barrier of one hundred years old.

Life expectancy has increased in recent years, while the population between 15 and 39 years old and children under 5 years old have decreased.

Centenarians are less exceptional and, in some cities, have already reached a considerable number. The population of older people is increasing and this will force us to reform labor and social protection laws, if we want to continue in the welfare state.

China boasts of having the largest number of elderly people. In fact, the International Medical and Nature Association (INMA) named the city of Nantong as "Longevity Capital" due to the number of centenarians residing there, a total of 1,031. The problem is that the majority of centenarians do not receive state aid and have financial problems. Maybe it's that some governments don't like the existence of older people.

The Okinawa archipelago also accumulates a good number of centenarians and of a total of 1.3 million people, 740 exceed the century of life. This fact would be due to a good state of health and, apparently, to their diet based on fish, whole grains, soy and, especially, vegetables. However, as we will see throughout this book, diet, while important, is not the key to longevity.

Mexico City, one of the busiest places on the American continent, has 1,103 registered people who are between 100 and 115 years of age, mostly women (72%), although only 410 receive the Alimony Pension for Seniors who by right corresponds to them.

We also know that there are 465,000 people over 80 years old. The majority of these people suffer from osteoarthritis and systemic hypertension, but there are few cases of cancer, as well as respiratory and cardiovascular problems and situations of anemia and obesity.

A little further north, in the state of Florida, is where there are the greatest number of long-lived people in the US. The warm climate and low cost of living make this town an attractive place to retire, along with low taxes and the discounts that can be enjoyed in food stores and others, as well as the numerous events that are organized in this great city for the elderly.

The idea is to promote active aging through the social participation of the elderly, an increase in their autonomy and the promotion of healthy behaviors.

Finally, in 2015, for example, there were 679 people aged 100 or over living in Wales. Sardinia, which has the highest number of centenarians in the world, has six centenarians for every 3,000 people.

Evolution of centenarians

In general, the secret to these people's longevity centers around social and emotional factors, such as expressing love, cultivating strong family and social ties, and participating in their community. Medical science, once it has assumed the deterioration of aging, can seriously hinder people's longevity.

Additionally, centenarians overwhelmingly cite loneliness and dependency as the most important issues that need to be controlled. Paradoxically, they suffer less from heart disease, stroke, and high blood pressure than the rest of the population. It is clear that if we take care of them a little, they will die of old age, that is, at 120 years old or more.

After the age of 100, aging slows down

Israeli doctor NirBarzilai of the Institute for Aging Research at the Albert Einstein College of Medicine in New York said:

"The usual recommendations for having a healthy life - not smoking, not drinking, getting plenty of exercise, eating a well-balanced diet, maintaining a low weight - work for young people, the average population, but not for the elderly. Centenarians belong to a separate class."

We must take this into account and focus more on the emotional level, on integration into society instead of isolation in residences, on the empowerment of the spiritual part, understanding as such the integration with the Whole, with the Source. When asked, most centenarians do not feel their chronological age; On average, they say they feel 20 years younger. Only their ID card reminds them of their chronological age.

Also, they are likely to have a positive attitude, are patient and tolerant, optimistic about simple things, enthusiasm for life, and a good sense of humor. As one centenarian in Sardinia cheerfully noted, the secret to living to 100 is "not to die before that."

For young people, aging is terrible, but they associate it with decrepitude, loss of bodily beauty and pain due to unresolved illnesses. But the essential thing is in the mind and emotions, the body is the vehicle in which we travel, but the drivers are us. If we want to have a good life, it is up to us.

The emotions

So we come to a key point in aging or change, as I prefer to define the passage of time. Personality is what is important, the vision of the world, everything more important than genetics, diet or exercise, three factors that are overly valued.

There is a clear tendency towards depression and, even more so, dissatisfaction with life, generating serious psychiatric problems. Society, turned into an eternal victim, blames others for its incorrect living, forgetting that the decision to adopt a healthy lifestyle corresponds to oneself.

People with correct emotions age (change) differently, more slowly. Finally, they die perhaps from similar diseases, but 30 years later, slowly releasing their vital breath.

The current food

Because we call it "junk food" so much, we have believed it and thus there is no way to assimilate it well; There is an emotional rejection that translates into an organic rejection. If we believe that it is not correct, it will harm us.

It should be noted that our diet has undergone enormous changes, just in approximately the last 50 years, and for many it has been for the worse. That fatalism is not correct. A person who is now celebrating her 100th birthday grew up with a very different diet from what a child who was born today, or even two decades ago, eats. But, although quality is considered more important than quantity, we must change this order: in the West we eat too much, especially at dinner time. "The graves are full of great dinners," says the wise saying. At the beginning of the 20th century, most people ate a large meal once a day and thanked fate – or God – that they could eat it. The body and mind united with the same goal: feeding.

The current public dietary guidelines are not correct; they always say the same clichés full of errors. The population is following wrong guidelines. "You have to eat everything", "meat two or three times a week", "fruit away from meals", "not drinking water during meals" and "five small meals are better than three"; So there is no way to be well nourished. They are doing great harm by leading the entire population down the wrong path when it comes to proper dietary choices.

These guidelines have even had international consequences, as nations that do not have the resources or scientific expertise to interpret the data simply model their own guidelines based on those of wealthy states.

In 1965, people in the United States got about 40% of their calories from carbohydrates, and another 40% of their calories came from fat. We have 20% left for proteins, too little for macronutrients in which lies the secret to longevity. Without sufficient proteins, without amino acids, body tissues, including nervous tissue and the chromosomes themselves, are not restored, they slowly deteriorate.

The 1980 guidelines urged eating a low-fat, high-carbohydrate diet; and in 2010, Americans had decreased their fat intake to less than 35 percent and increased their carbohydrate intake from 55 to 65 percent. Since then, this misguided recommendation to consume a diet based on carbohydrates and low in saturated fat, has been devastating. Believing that saturated fats are an enemy to avoid is as incorrect as claiming that we need to eat meat to meet our demands for vitamin B12. Specifically, saturated fats increase the amount of LDL cholesterol in large particles, never associated with heart problems, and, in the same way, they increase the amount of HDL cholesterol. Also, they help the metabolism and deposit of fat-soluble vitamins, A, D, E and K.

And regarding B12, we will insist on two common errors: despite being water-soluble, it maintains a stable deposit in the liver that is not easily eliminated.

And regarding its synthesis we must remember that it is made thanks to the help of the intestinal flora, the intrinsic factor of the stomach and the trace element cobalt. It is not necessary, therefore, to eat meat.

Transgenic foods

This is a controversial point, since GMOs are blamed for harming the health of humanity. But we have had them there since 1995, the year in which the first crop resistant to herbicides and some pests was approved.

To clarify the concepts, we will say that transgenesis is the horizontal transmission of genetic information, the deliberate administration of genetic material to correct a genetic problem or to provide cells with a new function. It would be, in principle, a laudable attempt to improve something.

It can be done to modify and improve descendants, in this case food, by changing a piece of DNA, thus changing only the affected cells, never the entirety. For example, the CRISPR/Cas9 technique (Clustered Regularly Interspaced Short Palindromic Repeats) which consists of inserting or cutting DNA using nuclease enzymes that will be repaired, or also inserting new DNA. That is, they manage to program the system to go to a specific position of any DNA (not just viral) and cut it. This tool can be used to regulate gene expression, label specific sites in the genome in living cells, identify and modify gene functions, and correct defective genes. The problem is that this RNA can hybridize, join with more than one site in the genome, which would lead the Cas9 enzyme to cut into a site that does not interest us.

Mathus, a British economist, developed the theory of population, published in his book Essay on the Principle of Population (1798), in which he explained that the population tends to grow faster than the supply of food available for its needs.

When there is an increase in food production greater than population growth, the growth rate is stimulated; On the other hand, if the population increases too much in relation to food production, growth slows down due to famines, diseases and wars. He predicted an inevitable famine due to the demographic growth of the population, just as it is now. They say about longevity, but they were wrong. The problem is not the amount of food available, but the distribution of wealth.

It was subsequently estimated that to obtain food for the 9.6 billion people that are expected to exist in 2050, it is necessary:

-Use new substances

-Reduce production costs

-New and greater quantity of raw materials

-Achieve better plant phenotypes that adapt to external circumstances

- Increase performance
- Improve productivity
- Improve agronomic characteristics.

Transgenic plants are characterized by:
- Resistance to herbicides, that is, phytosanitary products used to eliminate unwanted plants or interfering with the growth of weeds.
- Insect resistance.

Some of the problems currently detected:
- Antibiotic resistance
- Androsterility
- A biased and hostile public opinion
- The difficulty of introducing the transgenic gene only in the gene that we want to eliminate.

Regarding animal transgenics, we know that it is used for:
- Produce milk proteins
- Transplant organs from animals (pig) to humans.

Long-lasting diet

In terms of nutrition, today's centenarians have had a clear and obvious advantage. To put it more directly, they were not raised with forced or chemical-filled crops, nor do they suffer from dietary restrictions.

During the first 50 or 60 years of their lives – in which we are also included – they consumed whole foods, although when it comes to creating a basis for health, close provenance and correct handling (collection, packaging, distribution), they are also decisive.

Perhaps that is why there is so little divergence - in terms of specific dietary choices - to be found among centenarians. Now most of them say that they consume a little of everything (I insist on "a little"), including homemade sweets and foods that we usually avoid, such as meat and eggs. Perhaps the secret is in the environment in which they eat, not so much in the type of food.

Historically significant places

Sardinia

In Sardinia, which has the highest percentage of centenarians in the world (21 centenarians in a population of 10,000), to this day, there are no large processed food stores, no takeaways or fast food restaurants, Households grow their own fruits and vegetables, and the food is always prepared fresh, from scratch. There is hardly any food from distant overseas lands.

Another clue is that this type of locality requires them to walk every day, and much of the area has steep up or down paths, hills and cobblestone slopes. In addition, the culture of Sardinia favors socialization, which is another important factor, perhaps the most important, for longevity. They do not practice individualism, but social communication.

Puerto Rico

An attempt to modify the diet of the inhabitants of Puerto Rico, introducing beef from Argentina, resulted in an immediate decrease in the fertility of its people. However, when the opposite was done with the Eskimos and their traditional ration of seal meat and saturated fats was reduced, replaced by legumes and cereals, their birth rate tripled.

This leads us to a very interesting conclusion, as it indicates that in nature the survival of species predominates above all, a factor that is strongly linked to the health of individuals.

Caucasus

The inhabitants of the Caucasus have always had a reputation for being strong, good horsemen and effective lovers of women, and they frequently exceed one hundred years of age. When they reach the age of ninety they still want to remarry, they work four hours a day and they even dare to go hunting.

An important factor is that they do not need to work to survive, since the government assures them a decent pension and this means that they only dedicate themselves to doing those jobs that they like the most.

In these regions, obesity is not known and their caloric regime barely exceeds two thousand calories, even in times of cold or great activity. They eat vegetables and fruits all year round, meat only once a week, they do not eat soups or broths and they are never short of tomatoes, cucumbers, chives and garlic. They generously use herbs, both to season their meals and to heal themselves, and their daily ration of fruits is basically composed of apples, persimmons, pomegranates and grapes.

Continuing with the search for which is the key food, we know that their fat intake comes from walnuts (70 percent fat), which ensures a large and considerable amount of polyunsaturated and saturated fats. They don't try white sugar, which they replace with honey, which is much more nutritious and healthy. They do not like to drink tea or coffee and, however, they drink a wine made by themselves with very low alcohol content, although on cold days they frequently use vodka.

Hunza

Another highly healthy town is the state of Hunza, located in the Himalayas, whose inhabitants were immortalized in the novel *Lost*

Horizons, a story that was later made into a film by Frank Capra. According to Prince Mohammed Khan, the emir's brother, the secret of his long life lies in the daily ingestion of dried apricots, which contain the precious vitamin B15 or pangamic acid, incredibly prohibited in some countries.

Located at more than two thousand four hundred meters of altitude, the inhabitants of Hunza live in mud and stone houses and have a political regime that is not very democratic, although with soft laws.

The average age of its inhabitants exceeds ninety years and it is common to find elderly people up to one hundred and twenty years old, although the Government insists on altering the birth certificates of these people, so that the rest of the world stops be interested in them.

As I said before, apricots form the basis of their diet and they even eat crushed almonds.

They only eat meat in the cold winter months, they eat abundant fruits and vegetables, they drink very pure water from the glaciers and they take long daily walks.

Coffee and tea are replaced by apricot juice and children suck on apricot kernels as a substitute for candy.

The curious thing about this food is that Western experts have always prohibited the consumption of apricot kernels, claiming that it contains an appreciable amount of *cyanide*, precisely what gives it its bitter taste.

But what they have not explained is that the presence in our body of *beta-glucosidase* inactivates the toxicity of this organic cyanide and that the fleshy part of the fruit contains an enzyme called *rhodonase*, which compensates for the excesses of cyanide in the almond.

However, continued consumption of the nut can lead to health problems.

Vilcabamba

Continuing with our world tour we arrive at the Vilcabamba valley, located five hundred kilometers from Quito (Ecuador), where women frequently reach one hundred and twenty years of age and continue giving birth even at fifty years of age. Their pace of life is similar to the other two towns and consists of a diet of no more than two thousand calories a day, gentle but continuous work, clean air and water, as well as a preferably vegetarian diet. It is curious that none of the healthiest peoples focus their diet on meat.

About two thousand people live in this town and another three thousand more on the slopes, increasing significantly during the tourist season. Its temperature barely varies from 20°, except at nights when it gets a little cold. As in other towns, their houses are built with simple materials, mud and stones, and all their kitchen utensils are made with mud and none contain harmful metals.

Their consumption of herbs is high and there is no shortage of mint and orange leaves, with which they make infusions that replace coffee. The diet is essentially composed of cheese, fruits and vegetables, mainly papaya, corn, banana, barley, grapes, tomatoes and oats. They take the sugar natural, unrefined, from sugar cane.

About two thousand people live in this town and another three thousand more on the slopes, increasing significantly during the tourist season. Its temperature barely varies from 20°, except at nights when it gets a little cold. As in other towns, their houses are built with simple materials, mud and stones, and all their kitchen utensils are made with mud and none contain harmful metals.

Their consumption of herbs is high and there is no shortage of mint and orange leaves, with which they make infusions that replace coffee. The diet is essentially composed of cheese, fruits and vegetables, mainly papaya, corn, banana, barley, grapes, tomatoes and oats. They take the sugar natural, unrefined, from sugar cane.

This town does not know obesity or baldness, and men are capable of making love well into their nineties, something that fills them with pride. For many, the secret of such long life and fertility lies in a root called cassava, similar to potatoes, which they eat boiled daily.

Conclusion

These three towns that we have mentioned have some highly clarifying points in common:

> 1. They exercise daily without rushing; They don't compete, they just move and work
>
> 2. They barely eat animal meat
>
> 3. They consume freshly picked fruits and vegetables
>
> 4. Your caloric intake is never more than two thousand calories
>
> 5. They hardly drink alcohol or coffee, although they make their own spirits
>
> 6. They make abundant use of medicinal plants
>
> 7. They do not eat refined sugar or white flour
>
> 8. They live in places where pollution is unknown
>
> 9. They do not have to compete with other towns.

And the consumption of animal protein?

Here we are already beginning to scientifically dismantle the myth that we need to consume animal proteins. Furthermore, when analyzing animal meat we see that livestock, including pigs and sheep, transmit a type of sugar called Neu5Gc, which the immune system recognizes as foreign, when their meat is consumed. There is significant data that suggests that when the immune system Being exposed to this molecule, which comes from red meat, stimulates the development of an antibody to the lining of your own blood vessels.

Defenders of a meat diet maintain that meat is essential to provide protein, since it has greater biological value, that is, its richness in essential amino acids is greater than vegetables. This theory, maintained since the 19th century due to the subjective vision of a researcher named Liebing, has caused a lot of damage and I think that no one has bothered to disprove it.

It is true that certain vegetables contain a lower wealth of essential amino acids than meat, but this does not apply to the rest of the natural products. To give an example of some foods whose richness in essential amino acids is higher than meat, we have: soy, wheat germ, pollen, royal jelly, brewer's yeast, sesame seeds, millet and a long etc.

Furthermore, the combination of vegetables with cereals, tubers or legumes, finally provides a biological value equal to meat, without forgetting the greater net utility of protein, that is, the possibility that our body can metabolize it. In this sense, plant proteins have, for humans, a much higher net utility.

Active life and social support

Finding no specific dietary influence (apart from the fact that they have consumed whole foods for most of their lives), what other factor is at work in the longevity of these people?

In interviews and surveys carried out with centenarians, the following themes predominated:

> Keep a positive attitude and a sense of humor

> Have a strong social network from family and friends

> Do moderate exercise, but regular (for example, walking, riding a bicycle, gardening and swimming)

> Have a healthy life (No Smoking, or drink alcohol, etc.)

> Not have physical dependence

> Have faith/spirituality, and a sense of purpose in the life

> Stay mentally active and always learning something new

> Have a positive lifestyle (continued), integrated into society

In fact, the importance of having emotional social support has been scientifically verified, which is the factor that most centenarians give importance to for their longevity.

They do not ask for physical help so much as to continue feeling integrated into society.

An American meta-analysis of published studies found that having strong social support, in which the elderly felt needed by society, was positioned as the main factor determining longevity and survival. This factor, that of non-social exclusion, exceeds the influence of weight and even eclipses the influence of smoking.

Joy for the present

Happiness is another factor. Research confirms that people who are happy have greater longevity and live 35% longer lives. So it's no surprise that centenarians are a happy and optimistic bunch.

Apparently, somehow, having positive thoughts and attitudes has a powerful effect on the body that strengthens the immune system, boosts healthy emotions, reduces pain and provides stress relief. Curiously, the desire to help provides more satisfaction than the need to be helped.

In fact, it has been scientifically proven that happiness could have an impact on gene expression. A team of UCLA researchers showed that people who have a deep sense of happiness and well-being had lower levels of inflammatory gene expression, as well as a stronger antiviral and antibody response.

Likewise, while some of their longevity may depend on the DNA they were born with, an even greater part depends on epigenetics, over which they can exert great control.

Your diet, physical activity, environmental exposures, thoughts and emotions exert an epigenetic influence at every moment of the day, playing a fundamental role in aging and disease.

Money and longevity

There is a belief that money, while it does not necessarily lead to happiness, can lead to great longevity. After all, life is more comfortable with a good house, food, good doctors and entertainment. If you have great financial solvency, you could buy all the things that will provide you with health - they say -. Let's review the longevity of the rich and we will see that this is not the case.

On the contrary, living a "hard" life; That is, a life where physical activities are carried out, sometimes hard work, preferably outdoors, is something that most centenarians have in common.

Growing and/or eating fresh food, socializing with family and friends, appreciating life in general, and developing a sense of purpose—a reason to get up every morning—are other commonalities that centenarians share, no matter where they live. If we add to this a clear conscience and a desire to do good, we are already on the path to longevity.

Be sitting

According to recent research, if people reduced the amount of time they spend sitting, they could increase the years of their life expectancy.

Unfortunately, most people spend much of their day in a sitting position. It's hard to avoid these days, as working in front of a computer predominates, as does watching television, socializing and eating while sitting. In addition, most spend many hours a week traveling to and from work, something that is initially unrewarding.

The study estimates that reducing the average time we spend sitting to less than three hours a day could increase our life expectancy by two years. There aren't many, really, but at least we know that reducing the time we spend watching television helps us stay healthy. And the human being is bipedal, and we are designed to walk upright and rest lying down. We are one of the few species that sits very often, too often. The chair, furthermore, is not man's best invention, anatomically speaking.

In a study conducted at the Pennington Biomedical Research Center in Baton Rouge, Los Angeles, sedentary behaviors were determined to be an important risk factor similar to smoking and obesity.

Other studies have found that our sitting culture may be responsible for about 173,000 cases of cancer each year.

Because Western adults on average sit between 4.5 and five hours a day, a significant change in population-wide behavior would be needed to have an effect on life expectancy. This could be achieved through changes in the workplace, such as the use of standing desks and watching less television... However, we must consider the time we spend sitting eating, a position that also does not facilitate the journey of food through intestinal transit. Remember the carvings depicting people eating in ancient Rome and Greece, and you will know what the correct posture is.

To put this in perspective, the authors compared it to smoking, with each cigarette reducing life expectancy by almost 11 minutes.

If this cigarette is smoked after eating, sitting or watching television, the figure is certainly worrying.

Overall, researchers found that adults who spend an average of six hours watching television will reduce their life expectancy by just under 5 years, compared to someone who doesn't watch television. It doesn't seem like much, but if we add it to smoking and frequent stressful situations, the years lost are many.

The point is that sitting/watching television has an impact on mortality that is not insignificant and given the high prevalence of these behaviors in the population, there could be a notable reduction in the life expectancy of the population in general.

A recently published study looking at 800,000 people found that those who sat for longer periods of time were twice as likely to have diabetes or heart disease compared to those who spent less time sitting.

According to researcher Thomas Yates, MD, even for people who are active in other ways, sitting for long periods of time appears to be a risk factor for diseases such as diabetes, cardiovascular disease and kidney disease.

Emotional balance and optimism

In a study of 100 older adults (average 81 years old), people who were exposed to positive implicit messages (words like creative, active, and fit) experienced benefits in their physical strength.

It is evident that the mind has power over the body and all these centenarians exemplify it. If you think that your mind and body deteriorate as you age, then that will happen.

But the opposite is also true, specifically if your positive mindset is combined with the basic requirements for a healthy life (non-hostile positive thinking, sleeping well, staying active, and eating right).

Most centenarians say they feel 20 years younger than their chronological age and their mentality has a lot to do with their self-perception. It is possible that if biological age were evaluated it would be very similar to what they feel.

Centennials and food

Most centenarians tend to eat food they grow themselves or produce from nearby lands. However, and this is a factor that must be taken into account, the environment surrounding the moment of eating must be rewarding, free of distortion or aggressiveness. With which we can understand that perhaps the environment where you eat is more important than the food itself.

Emma Morano, who at 117 was the oldest person in the world (now deceased), told the media that one of her diet secrets was to eat three eggs (two of them raw) and raw ground beef every day. I suppose this will greatly disappoint those who defend a vegetarian diet as the best option, but it confirms the idea that I have raised previously: what is important is the environment and how you receive the food, more than the food itself. What we don't know is how many years Emma would have lived if she had also eaten healthy foods.

In addition to what they eat, many centenarians also mentioned the importance of intermittent fasting, not overeating, and eating once a day. What we already know is that eating three times a day, and in between small amounts, is a clear error that some wrong doctors advise.

Stable relationships, fond memories and living in the moment

Any aspect in common between centenarians? Stable and positive relationships. Each spoke fondly of their marriages even though their respective partners had died decades ago, and even though they had divorced them; Everyone still had very fond memories. Why not remember better the pleasant moments that have always existed? It is important to remember life experiences and relationships with appreciation and gratitude.

In fact, the researchers found a 50% increase in the likelihood of survival in participants with more stable social relationships. Although material possessions provide well-being, they are not always linked to the feeling of feeling happy. What's more, the "newness" of possessions disappears, as does the joy they bring, but pleasurable emotional experiences increase the feeling of vitality and "feeling alive" during the experience and when remembering it.

Additionally, most centenarians, regardless of their health status, tend to have positive attitudes, optimism, and enthusiasm for life. It is important to live in the present, not to think about what has been lost, but to appreciate everything that has been done (and remains to be done).

It's also worth mentioning, that none of them are planning to leave anytime soon.

Each one talks about feeling strong and hopes to continue living each day to the fullest. They are active - physically, mentally and socially. This also helps them stay young and healthy.

Help, rather than ask for help

The willingness to help other people also gives a sense of purpose and can even produce the so-called "helper's feeling of happiness," which could occur because doing good releases feel-good hormones, such as oxytocin, while reducing the levels of stress hormones such as cortisol.

Personality traits also affect longevity, which could also play an important role in centenarians. For example, having a sense of purpose and feeling productive have been shown to promote longevity.

Consciousness, specifically, was defined as a marker for longevity. Researchers believe the reason for this is that conscious behavior influences other behaviors. For example, conscious people tend to make healthier choices, have work they enjoy, and have life partners they are happy with. Conscientious people also tend to be more productive, even after they retire, and tend to see their work as having a purpose.

Being a Lifelong Learner and having a natural curiosity about life and a desire to continue learning likely also play a role in the longevity connection.

Despite all of the above, it seems that there is no pattern to being long-lived. The usual recommendations for a healthy life - not smoking, not drinking, exercising, eating naturally and keeping weight under control - which are recommended for everyone, do not work for centenarians. It seems that its energy comes from within itself.

They, the long-lived, advise us to always do the right thing, to be independent, to not ask for help and rather to give it, to be kind to others, show them respect and help them whenever possible. Furthermore, they insistently advise us not to take medications.

The data is sobering and we know that there are between 96,000 and 105,000 centenarians living in the United States and about 12,640 in the United Kingdom. Research indicates that the number of American centenarians has doubled every decade since 1950, and it is expected that by 2050, the number of centenarians living in the United States will exceed one million. There are about 65 verified super centenarians alive today, but an unofficial number put numbers as high as 3,507. In Spain there are 14,487 centenarians, according to data from the latest registry of the National Institute of Statistics (INE), more than double the number in 2000.

Happiness and epigenetics

Happy people live longer than 35 percent, according to one study.

Another study found that happiness and joy improve health and increase longevity, and obviously, optimistic people live longer than pessimistic people, so it's no surprise that centenarians are a happy and optimistic group of people.

Positive thoughts and attitudes somehow seem to do things in the body that strengthen the immune system, increase positive emotions, decrease pain, and relieve stress. In fact, it has been scientifically proven that happiness can alter your genes.

A team of UCLA researchers showed that people with a deep sense of happiness and well-being had lower levels of inflammatory gene expression and a stronger antibody and antiviral response.

This falls into the realm of epigenetics—changing the way genes work, turning them on and off.Part of your longevity may depend on the DNA you were born with, but more of it depends on epigenetics—over which you have greater control. Your thoughts, feelings, emotions, diet and other lifestyle factors influence every minute of the day, playing the main role in aging and disease. Maybe it is not so important to avoid ice cream even if we are told it is harmful, since He feels happy eating it, at least once in a while.

However, they should know that happiness requires effort, it never comes from outside.

CHAPTER 4

TELOMERES

The discovery of Telomeres

Telomeres constitute specialized structures that form the ends of eukaryotic chromosomes that participate in cellular functions as important as mitosis, chromosomal stability and the lifespan of cell lines. Recently, its relationship with some diseases, especially cancer, has been demonstrated. During the last 2 decades, much progress has been made in the knowledge of its structure and dynamics.

They were identified by Hermann J. Muller during the 1930s and for this he received the Nobel Prize in Physiology and Medicine in 1946. Since then, knowledge of these structures has deepened extraordinarily, thanks to the introduction of modern Molecular Genetics technology. A summary of the main works carried out in the first years of application of these techniques was published in 1984 by Blackburn and Szostack.

In the 1950s, scientists who barely understood how genes are copied observed that when a cell is about to divide, DNA molecules, which contain the four bases that make up the genetic code, are copied, base by base. , thanks to the enzyme DNA polymerase.

However, in each of the two strands of DNA, the final part cannot be copied. Therefore, chromosomes appeared to shorten each time a cell divided, which does not always happen. The discovery of telomeres and the associated enzyme solved the problem: telomeres protected chromosomes.

In the 1970s, as the mechanisms behind DNA replication became better understood, it became clear that DNA polymerase, the enzyme responsible for DNA replication, could not completely synthesize the end of linear DNA. In 1972, James Watson called this the ultimate replication problem. At about the same time, in a Moscow subway station, Alexey Olovnikov also recognized Watson's problem in an analogy between the train tracks representing DNA and the train representing DNA polymerase. However, Olovnikov went further by proposing that the eventual replication problem would result in the shortening of telomeres with each round of replication and that, because DNA was replicated during cell division, this mechanism could be the cause of the replicative senescence (RS). Soon after, studies by Leonard Hayflick and colleagues found that the nucleus controls SR.

It was known that DNA polymerase requires an RNA primer to start synthesis in the correct direction. At the end of a linear chromosome, DNA polymerase can synthesize the leading strand to the end of the chromosome.

However, on the lagging strand, DNA polymerase synthesis relies on a series of fragments, called Okazaki, each of which requires an RNA primer. Without DNA to serve as a template for a new primer, the replication machinery is unable to synthesize the sequence complementary to the final primer event. The result is an end-replication problem in which the sequence is lost in each round of DNA replication. Olovkikov's model turned out to be incredibly accurate.

Later, Barbara McClintock (Nobel Prize 1983), had observed that the structures formed at the ends of chromosomes, telomeres, prevented chromosomes from adhering to each other. Its protective role resembled the myelin sheath.

Elizabeth Blackburn, Australian biochemist, discoverer of telomerase, studying the chromosomes of Tetrahymena, a ciliated unicellular organism, identified a DNA sequence that was repeated several times at the ends of the chromosomes. The function of this sequence, CCCCAA, was clear. Simultaneously, Jack Szostak had made the observation that a linear DNA molecule, a type of minichromosome, was rapidly degraded when introduced into yeast cells.

Blackburn presented his results at a conference in 1980 and they soon interested Jack Szostak and Blackburn and decided to perform an experiment whose results were published in 1982.

The DNA sequence of the telomeres protected the minichromosomes from degradation, through a fundamental mechanism not previously recognized . Later, it became evident that telomere DNA with its characteristic sequence is present in most plants and animals, from amoeba to man.

The miracle enzyme

Carol Greider, supervised by Blackburn, began to investigate whether the formation of telomere DNA could be due to an unknown enzyme. In 1984, Greider discovered signs of enzymatic activity in a cell extract, an enzyme, which they called telomerase, carrying RNA as well as proteins. The RNA component turned out to contain the sequence CCCCAA, the template when building the telomere, while the protein component is required for the construction work, i.e. enzymatic activity. Telomerase extends the DNA at the telomeres, providing a platform that allows DNA polymerases to copy the entire length of the chromosome without losing the end portion.

Telomeric DNA

In almost all eukaryotes studied, telomeric DNA (tDNA) consists of clustered repeats of small nucleotide sequences. The length of the telomere is variable and each organism has a characteristic average length, as does the amount of tDNA per chromosome. In some organisms, the average telomere length responds to genetic, epigenetic or nutritional changes.

Telomeric DNA consists of small repeat sequences rich in guanine bases, with a monofibrillar end that can form secondary type structures by pairing of guanine bases.

These repeats serve for protein binding, both in the double strand and in the monofibrillar zone. The more telomeric sequences are known, the more difficult it is to find a consensus sequence. The existence of multiple telomeric sequences suggests that telomere functions do not require a single sequence. The finding of telomeric sequences in internal sites of the chromosomes demonstrates that they by themselves do not make telomeres.

Telomere shortening is now considered the main causal mechanism of SR and telomere length is the molecular clock that counts accumulated cell population doublings (CPDs) and what cells can support. Although it was previously known that telomere shortening occurs with every subculture, the key finding linking telomeres to RS was made in 1998 by scientists at the Geron Corporation.

The studies have been carried out mainly on ciliates, single-celled microscopic organisms, which are generally found in the plankton of rivers, lakes, seas and oceans, whose macronuclei can contain from 40,000 to 1,000,000 telomeres depending on the species, so they constitute a excellent source of telomeric components and the enzymes that participate in its replication.

Subsequently, it has been proven that the aspects described in ciliates are present in other organisms. In mammals, where they are much longer, they are made up of nucleosomes, but towards the most extreme area they appear as telosomas. This shows that at least in part there is structural conservation of the telomeres. They also show somewhat surprising differences in other species.

Telomeres delay cell aging

Scientists have investigated what role the telomere might play in the cell, and one of the experiments identified yeast cells with mutations that resulted in a gradual shortening of telomeres. These cells grew little and eventually stopped dividing.

Blackburn and his co-workers made mutations in telomerase RNA and observed similar effects in Tetrahymena, ciliated protozoa found in fresh waters. In both cases, this led to premature cellular aging and senescence. In contrast, intact telomeres prevented chromosomal damage and delayed cellular senescence. Later, Greider's group showed that the senescence of human cells is also delayed by telomerase. Research in this area has been intense and it is now known that the DNA sequence at the telomere attracts proteins that form a protective cap around the fragile ends of the DNA strands.

These discoveries had a great impact on the scientific community and many scientists speculated that telomere shortening could be the reason for aging, not only in individual cells, but also in the organism as a whole. But the aging process has turned out to be complex and is now believed to depend on several different factors, although the telomere is one of them, and epigenetics, let's not forget.

Human cells have a different division cycle, with the intestinal, stomach, bone marrow and skin being the fastest, while the latest are the bone, heart and liver. Paradoxically, it will be on the slow renewal cells that we will be able to act most effectively, since telomere repair takes time.

In contrast, cancer cells have the ability to divide infinitely and yet retain their telomeres. The reason? They activate their own telomerase, regardless of the state of the organism in which they develop. Even in seriously damaged human organisms, cancer cells can remain in optimal condition.

How, then, to escape cellular senescence? Perhaps we should copy the survival mechanism that malignant cells have to increase telomerase activity. Stress control could be the key.

Consequently, it has been proposed that cancer could be treated by eradicating telomerase from these cells. Several studies are underway in this area, including clinical trials evaluating vaccines targeting cells with inherited diseases. But we don't like vaccines, because they deceive the immune system.

Defects in telomerase are known to be especially prominent in diseases such as congenital aplastic anemia, in which insufficient cell divisions in the stem cells of the bone marrow lead to severe anemia. Certain inherited diseases of the skin and lungs are also caused by telomerase defects.

Telomeres and cancer

In previous paragraphs we have explained that telomeres determine how cells can duplicate, and therefore links have been established with the aging process and cancer, in terms of cell suicide. In repeated mitosis, the telomeres become shorter and the cell stops dividing and ends up causing apoptosis, preventing renewal. However, those cells with defects in the signaling pathway, such as tumor cells, continue to replicate relentlessly.

When researchers analyzed the mechanism of cell death, they saw that telomeres were much more decisive than previously thought when it came to stopping cancer. Mitosis was found to be longer in cells approaching suicide. That is, instead of the 30-45 minutes it normally lasts, these cells have mitosis that lasts 2 to 20 hours or more.

The reason for this, they explain, is that the telomeres have lost a protein that is key when it comes to initiating the self-destruction process. Using real-time images of cells, they found that a type of cellular stress, called telomere fusion, could cause prolonged mitosis and eventually cell death. That is, the telomeres of the cells in this state lost their protective protein and activated the self-destruct sequence. And this process has nothing to do with the slow and steady accumulation of genomic instability.

In this sense, the finding is believed to open new avenues for understanding how cell growth and telomere fusions translate to the final phases of mitosis, suggesting possible implications of telomere biology in chemotherapy.

For example, some chemotherapy treatments, such as taxol for breast cancer, try to stop cancer by stopping mitosis, which prevents cancer cells from dividing. The researchers now hypothesize that it might be possible to improve these mitosis inhibitors, for example, by unprotecting telomeres to make cells more susceptible to drugs. It might also be possible to determine whether cells in a particular tumor have shorter or unprotected telomeres, and if so, the tumor would logically be much more sensitive to mitosis inhibitors. However, there is one fact that is often forgotten: tumor cells make and activate their own telomerase.

Generally inhibiting telomerase or deliberately shortening telomeres would cause general chromosome chaos.

Telomere replication

In replication, two DNA molecules are created, each composed of one strand of the original DNA and a new complementary strand. That is, the existing strands serve as a complementary mold for the new ones.

In the structure of telomeres, the area of repetitions in the double strand predominates and only the terminal end has the monofibrillar structure. Although telomerase is necessary to maintain telomere length, this enzyme only lengthens the G strand. Replication of the C strand must be done by the conventional polymerase system. In yeast, humans, and other organisms, telomeres replicate at the end of the S phase, during which the cell synthesizes a complete copy of DNA in its nucleus. It also duplicates a microtubule organization structure called the centrosome. As a consequence of this impediment, in each cycle of DNA replication the linear chromosomes undergo a small shortening. If this shortening is excessive, the integrity of the chromosome may be affected.

So telomere replication is necessary to compensate for the small, slow loss of DNA that results from incomplete replication, and should therefore be considered a repair function.

In this process, telomeric DNA does not exactly have the role of template.

The state of telomeres depends on several factors, including the production of telomerases, the frequency of their action on each particular telomere, and the rate of tDNA degradation.

Knowing that telomeres represent essential structures for cells, as they prevent chromosome fusion, maintaining their stability and participating in both meiosis and mitosis, we find another even more notable function, which is to serve as a mitotic clock that measures and regulates the number of cell divisions. Telomeres shorten with each cell division and the number of divisions the cell can undergo correlates with the length of the telomeres. This shortening could eliminate genes essential for life or silence nearby genes due to the telomere position effect. A critical length could be the signal for entry into cellular senescence.

However, it is worth insisting that it is not related to the age of the organism and its shortening can occur at any age.

Medical perspectives

The discovery of the unique nucleoprotein structure of telomeres and their structural and functional phylogenetic conservation demonstrate the essential nature of these structures for the life of the cell.

The existence of telomerases solves the old problem about the replication of the ends of linear DNA molecules, however, these findings raise new problems. Among them is determining the function of the tRNA in the area that does not function as a template and its possible participation in enzymatic catalysis, the chemical reactions they cause. It is also necessary to elucidate the factors that regulate the activity of the enzyme on the one hand and the length of the telomeres on the other, as well as the molecular mechanisms that link telomeres with the regulation of cell proliferation. The possible application of this knowledge for the diagnosis and treatment of proliferative diseases, especially cancer, will also be interesting and transcendental.

Using electron microscopy, it was revealed that telomeres are not linear, but instead appear to form duplex loops, called t-loops. Although not completely understood, the predominant hypothesis is that these loops stabilize or cap telomeres, thus protecting them, preventing DNA damage.

TRF2 (telomeric repeat binding factor 2), a human gene, protects telomeres and inhibition of TRF2 induces apoptotic cell death, while overexpression of TRF2 reduces the senescent checkpoint of cells in terms of cell length. telomeres. These results suggest that telomere coverage, not just telomere length, is crucial to avoiding telomere dysfunction and preventing cellular senescence. Results showing that telomerase disruption can slow cell proliferation and disrupt excess single-stranded telomeres without telomere shortening support this view. A plausible hypothesis is that telomere shortening may destabilize or even prevent telomere capping, leading to SR.

It is still under discussion whether the end-replication problem is responsible for telomere shortening. SR can occur in human fibroblasts in the absence of cell division and short telomeres. Cells remain confluent for long periods of time - up to 12 weeks - upon exiting the cell cycle. The small proportion of cells that continue to divide suffered less CPD (cancer of unknown primary origin) than normal, presumably due to compensatory cycling. Although quiescent cells do not appear to lose telomeres, the cells undergo accelerated telomere shortening after extended periods of confluency. Some research suggests that overhang erosion occurs in cellular senescence and is prevented by telomerase expression. The progressive erosion appears to be a result of cell division and not an effect of RS. However, the exact molecular mechanisms behind telomere shortening and dysfunction remain undetermined.

Since a normal human diploid cell contains 92 telomeres, another issue is whether it is the average telomere length or the shortest telomere that triggers RS.

Evidence in mice indicates that shorter telomeres are responsible for the induction of RS. However, a study in human fibroblasts found that the onset of RS shows a better correlation with the average telomere length than with the shortest telomere. Again, the controversy.

Telomeres and DNA damage

It is known that the early proteins E6 and E7 of HPV (human papillomavirus) alter cell growth by inactivating tumor suppressor proteins, such as p53, promoting the progression of premalignant to malignant lesions.

Telomere dysfunction causes an activation of DNA damage response pathways, such as an activation of p53 (transcription factor). Infection of human fibroblasts with viral oncogenes results in a prolonged replicative lifespan after which the cells enter a stage called crisis, during which the cells proliferate, but the proportion of cells entering apoptosis gradually increases and therefore Therefore, the number of cells eventually decreases, possibly due to extremely short telomeres. Sometimes, possibly with the help of epigenetic elements, immortal cells emerge from the crisis with stabilized telomeres, usually involving the activation of telomerase.

Overall, regardless of the changes that occur during telomere dysfunction, the mechanisms that trigger growth arrest appear to involve DNA damage pathways, and short telomeres lead to chromosomal fusions.

Strong physiological stimuli or prolonged stress stop cell growth, a state also called quiescence.

Finally, everything indicates that the study in mice related to telomeres is not extrapolated to humans, since the regulation of RS and the dysfunction in telomerase are different.

Aging, cancer and telomeres

The role of telomeres in SR has led to the suggestion that telomerase can be used as an anti-aging therapy, at least as stated by Fossel (1996), Blasco (2005), Shawi and Autexier (2008). However, as mentioned above, the relationship between SR and the aging of organisms is controversial.

As with the replicative potential (the ability to duplicate), telomere length in vivo is very heterogeneous as has been proven in liver cells, lymphocytes, skin cells, blood and colonic mucosa. For example, telomere shortening appears to impair immune T cell function and telomerase activators may restore a healthier functional profile. Other studies found weak correlations between donor age and telomere length, while some studies found no correlation at all. Long telomeres have been found in cells from centenarians.

Together, these results indicate that telomere length varies widely between individuals and between different tissues, and that their shortening can occur in some tissues in vivo in association with certain pathologies and with age; this is similar to what is observed for senescent cells. An association between telomere length and mortality has been observed in people aged 60 and older, and telomere shortening appears to accelerate in people living more stressful lives. Although these results support the idea that telomere shortening is a marker of stress and related pathologies, not everyone wants to relate it to aging, as occurs with Werner syndrome (premature aging).

Although average telomere length at birth does not correlate with longevity in birds, the rate of telomere shortening in erythrocytes has been reported to correlate with longevity in birds. When telomeres gradually shorten, cells from generation four animals show aneuploidy (e.g. trisomy of chromosome 21) and other chromosomal aberrations.

The abnormalities were observed in the third generation and the last generation animals showed some signs of accelerated aging. It is controversial whether these animals are aging more rapidly or simply developing a variety of pathologies.

Overall, these results suggest that telomerase activity could be crucial for the normal functioning of highly proliferative organs in mice. However, telomere length and/or telomerase activity alone do not explain why humans age more slowly than other primates and live much longer than mice.

On the other hand, in the frog Xenopus laevis, another animal with a slow aging rate, no large variation in telomere length has been observed. The way telomere length does not affect the lifespan of cloned animals is also at odds with the role of telomeres in aging.

Increased telomerase activity has been associated with skin malignancy as a result of exposure to ultraviolet radiation, which seems to indicate a defensive state of the organism. For some scientists, however, increased telomerase activity represents an increase in malignancy, not a defensive mechanism. Error of judgment, such as giving the increase in temperature in cases of infections a harmful role.

Senescent cells probably accumulate in some tissues and may contribute to organ dysfunction, but telomere mechanisms may play a more favorable role. Some aging-altering genetic interventions appear to influence tissue homeostasis by affecting senescence, cell proliferation, and cell death.

Evidence from genetic manipulation experiments on telomeric signal transduction indicated that it improves resistance against cancer but does not increase aging. It can be argued that the strongest evidence for telomerase's role in aging is that it appears to eliminate cancer. through improved expression of p53 and INK4a/ARF, and lengthening of life. Although the reasons for aging are unclear, these findings point toward some level of protection against age-related degeneration through optimization of pathways associated with telomeres and SR.

Families affected by hereditary dyskeratosis also have shortened telomeres. Features of dyskeratosis congenita include bone marrow failure, which is the most common cause of death, abnormal skin pigmentation, leukoplakia and nail dystrophy.

The role of stem cells has also been suggested. Judging from the phenotype of dyskeratosis congenita, telomeres are crucial in rapidly proliferating tissues. A study on telomere length suggests a causal role of short telomeres in heart disease and other age-related diseases, so some effects of telomere shortening on age-related diseases other than cancer, should be considered.

In conclusion, it is unquestionable that cellular senescence and telomere biology are important in cancer and may be suitable for developing cancer treatments and helping to understand human aging.

It is highly likely that cellular senescence, caused primarily by stress and telomere shortening, may contribute to aging and age-related diseases. In fact, a genetic variant of telomerase has been associated with longer telomeres and exceptional human longevity.

Protection from age-related heart diseases

Researchers link telomere length to resistance to age-related genetic diseases.

Scientists at the Gladstone Institute have identified a very important mechanism that protects people from human diseases linked to aging. This discovery also helps explain the chronicity and severity of diseases that typically occur in humans.

Scientists believe that telomere shortening in mice that have a genetic mutation is linked to heart disease, specifically, a buildup of calcium within the heart's vessels and valves. This model allows researchers to identify new medications for the disease, and could lead to solving other human aging disorders. The disease causes calcium to build up inside the heart until the aortic valve calcifies (CAVD) and hardens. The solution is to replace the valve through surgery. The disease develops with age and one of the two copies of the NOTCH1 gene suffers a mutation. Most people have two copies of these genes. When the first copy is lost, the remaining copy cannot create enough protein to allow it to function properly.

Gladstone scientists published the results of a recent study in the Journal of Clinical Research. These researchers associated telomere length with risk and resistance to diseases. The results show that telomere length plays a fundamental role in human disease that is age-dependent.

The model offers the opportunity to analyze the mechanisms through which telomeres impact disease and are age-dependent. The model also provides a means to test treatments for aortic valve disease.

To the researchers' surprise, mice with shortened telomeres and the NOTCH1 mutation showed the same cardiac abnormalities seen in humans, and mice with short telomeres suffered the most heart damage. Some even show signs of valve disease immediately after birth. Telomere length is thought to affect disease severity through alteration of gene expression.

It should be noted that previous research determined that people with valve calcification had shorter telomeres compared to healthy patients of a similar age. The new findings indicate that telomere length is responsible for differences in disease severity. The gradual shortening of long telomeres that serve as protection for the chromosome reproduces the disease caused by the NOTCH1 mutation and increases the severity of the disease in humans.

Gladstone scientists published the results of a recent study in the Journal of Clinical Research. These researchers associated telomere length with risk and resistance to diseases. The results show that telomere length plays a fundamental role in human disease that is age-dependent. The model offers the opportunity to analyze the mechanisms through which telomeres impact disease and are age-dependent.

The model also provides a means to test treatments for aortic valve disease.

To the researchers' surprise, mice with shortened telomeres and the NOTCH1 mutation showed the same cardiac abnormalities seen in humans, and mice with short telomeres suffered the most heart damage. Some even show signs of valve disease immediately after birth. Telomere length is thought to affect disease severity through alteration of gene expression.

It should be noted that previous research determined that people with valve calcification had shorter telomeres compared to healthy patients of a similar age. The new findings indicate that telomere length is responsible for differences in disease severity. The gradual shortening of long telomeres that serve as protection for the chromosome reproduces the disease caused by the NOTCH1 mutation and increases the severity of the disease in humans.

Accelerated telomere shortening in response to stress

Numerous studies demonstrate links between chronic stress and rates of poor health, including risk factors for cardiovascular disease and poor immune function. However, the exact mechanisms of how stress undermines health are dubious, essentially because stress is not an evil, but rather a coping mechanism.

The hypothesis is that stress affects health by modulating the rate of cellular aging.

Oxidation, overload and cell apoptosis are the most plausible conclusions. We found evidence that psychological stress, both perceived stress and chronicity of stress, are significantly associated with greater oxidative stress, lower telomerase activity, and shorter telomere length, known determinants of senescence and longevity. cell in peripheral blood mononuclear cells from healthy patients.

Premenopausal women, with the highest levels of perceived stress, have shorter telomeres on average, and a decade of additional aging, compared to women with low stress. These findings have implications for understanding how, at the cellular level, stress can promote the early onset of age-related diseases.

People who are stressed for long periods tend to show dark circles under their eyes, and psychological stress is commonly thought to lead to premature aging and related diseases, including risk factors for cardiovascular disease and worse immune function. However, the exact mechanisms of how this stress exerts these effects are not well known, including whether stress accelerates aging at the cellular level and how cellular aging translates into aging of the organism.

Research continues to point to the crucial role of telomeres and telomerase in cellular aging and potentially disease.

We remember that when cells divide, the telomere does not reproduce completely due to the limitations of DNA polymerases in completing the replication of the ends of linear molecules, which leads to its shortening with each repetition. When telomeres shorten significantly, the cell enters senescence and doubles its errors in mitosis.

In people, telomeres shorten with age in all replicating somatic cells that have been examined, including fibroblasts and leukocytes. Thus, telomere length can serve as a biomarker of a cell's biological, not chronological, age or potential for cell division.

Nutrition and telomeres

Nutritionists have long been interested in the dynamics of telomere lengthening in the body, and how telomeres figure into human health and lifespan. Although in 1973 Alexey Olovnikov said that as we age telomeres become shorter and therefore DNA replication and cell division cease completely, a growing body of research is showing that certain nutrients play a very important role in protecting of telomere length, greatly affecting lifespan.

For example, in a recent study, scientists found that folate, a component of the B vitamins, plays an important role in maintaining DNA integrity and methylation, which in turn influences telomere lengthening.

Researchers also found that women who took vitamin B12 supplements had longer telomeres than those who did not take it. Vitamin D3, zinc, iron, omega-3 fatty acids, and vitamins C and E also influence telomere length. This supports the conclusions of a previous study conducted in 2009, which provided the first epidemiological evidence that multivitamin use is associated with telomere lengthening in people.

Compared with people who did not take multivitamins, the relative lengthening of leukocyte DNA telomeres was on average 5.1% greater among people who took multivitamins daily. In the micronutrient analysis, increased intake of vitamins C and E from foods were associated with lengthened telomeres, even after adjusting for multivitamin use.

The mechanism by which nutrients appear to affect telomere length is by influencing the activity of telomerase, the enzyme that adds telomeric repeats to the ends of your DNA. There are certain diseases that, now, we know for sure depend on the good condition of the telomeres to be eradicated:

Decreased immune response against infections

Type 2 diabetes

Atherosclerotic lesions

Intestinal, testicular and splenic atrophy.

CHAPTER 5

THE ROLE OF TELOMERASE

Telomerase is a ribozyme that lengthens telomeres and thus corrects normal erosion. It has two components: an RNA component and a catalytic subunit (protein folding or binding). Telomerase activity parallels the expression of the catalytic subunit (hTERT-telomerase reverse transcriptase) and ectopic hTERT expression (expression of a gene in a tissue where it is not normally expressed), being sufficient to restore telomerase activity. in human cells. We must remember that HTERT is often upregulated in rapidly dividing cells, including both embryonic stem cells and adult stem cells. Since it lengthens the telomeres of stem cells, it increases the lifespan of these cells by allowing indefinite division without shortening the telomeres. Therefore, it is responsible for the self-renewal properties of stem cells.

Telomerase activity is decisive in immortal cell lines, although the definitive discovery came when it was demonstrated that the expression of hTERT in human cells prevents RS. Human fibroblasts immortalized with hTERT divide vigorously, show no markers of cellular senescence, and no signs of neoplastic transformation. Even expression of hTERT in late passage fibroblasts appears to reverse the loss of function characteristic of pre-senescent cells.

However, telomerase is not the only mechanism capable of lengthening telomeres, since good epigenetics is capable of modifying the tendency towards senescence. There are several immortal telomerase-negative cell lines with typically a wide variety of telomere lengths. Although the exact mechanisms behind what is called alternative telomere lengthening remain largely unknown, several recombination processes may be involved. However, whether using telomerase or not, all known immortal cell lines must stabilize their telomeres.

Single-celled eukaryotic cells must also stabilize their telomeres. For example, defects in telomere replication have been shown to trigger senescence in yeast.

hTERT expression

Although telomere length regulates RS (replicative senescence) and can be seen as a mitotic clock, the mechanisms involved are more complex than they may at first appear. We will now see a fairly detailed and technical analysis of the molecular mechanisms involved and later the potential role of telomeres and telomerase in aging and cancer.

We have already indicated that telomere length is neither the only nor the last cell timekeeper.

During telomerase immortalization of human cell lines, several researchers noticed that the immortalized cells had shorter telomeres than those controlled for growth. Surprisingly, these immortalized cells had fewer chromosome fusions, which are the most notable result of short telomeres. Similarly, it was observed in yeast that certain telomerase-negative strains aged more with longer telomeres than immortal telomerase-positive strains. Since telomere length alone could not explain these observations, other factors had to be involved.

Many human somatic tissues have no detectable telomerase activity, however, bone marrow and hematopoietic cells, among others, express telomerase. Furthermore, telomerase activity is highest in primitive progenitor cells and is then regulated during proliferation and differentiation. Other reports associate normally low levels of telomerase activity with human stem cells, although probably not mesenchymal (adult) stem cells, with the capacity to differentiate into various cell types. Telomerase activity has been detected in some highly proliferating normal human somatic cells, for example, in skin cells, immune system cells, and colorectal tissues. A decrease in telomerase activity was observed in blood mononuclear cells with age and human germ cells have been found to express hTERT.

Telomerase activity varies at different stages of life. It has been detected in ovaries and testes in fetuses, newborns and adults, but not in eggs or mature sperm. The blastocyst (embryo of 5 or 6 days of development after fertilization, prior to its implantation in the uterus) and most of the somatic tissues of 16 to 20 weeks of development, exhibit a high level of telomerase that disappears after birth.

It is also high in adult tissues with intense cell proliferation such as endothelial cells and the endometrium. In other cells it can be induced at certain stages of life, as occurs with the activation of T and B lymphocytes.

This function of telomeres immediately relates them to the transformation of a healthy cell into a cancerous one. In one of the first works on the subject, it was found that in cultured cells from 18 different human tissues, there was telomerase activity in 98% of the immortal ones and none in 22 mortal ones. Likewise, there was also activity in 90% of 100 biopsies from 12 types of tumors and none in 50 from normal somatic tissues.

Subsequent studies have confirmed increased telomerase activity in breast, prostate, astrocytomas and other cancers. These findings could have important clinical implications, although we should attack the aggressor and not the messenger.

The determination of telomerase activity could be used for the early diagnosis of cancer in non-invasive tests and selective inhibitors of the enzyme could be used as antitumor agents with a high degree of selectivity for transformed cells. However, as we will repeat several times, tumor cells do not depend on organic telomerase, as they produce and activate their own.

At the end of the day, they are trying to survive. Telomerase, in tumor pathologies, increases to stabilize organic functions, and decreases again when the cancer appears resolved. If not, continue increasing. Overexpression of telomerase does not favor the development of cancer, rather, it attempts to control it. A simile is when cholesterol levels increase, which for some scientists represents a serious danger, when in reality it is one of the best organic defenses to correct errors in hormone production and cell permeability.

Telomerase gene therapy in old mice also moderately increased lifespan and appears to have independent telomere lengthening functions, such as in protecting mitochondria under stress. Another study showed that reactivating telomerase reverses degeneration in mice.

During telomeric DNA replication, the "G-rich" helix is synthesized by telomerase, whose RNA component contains a sequence complementary to that of the telomeric repeat sequence, and can act as a terminal transferase.

Telomerase, as we know, adds the necessary telomeric DNA to the ends of the telomere, although it also has direct functions as a protector.

In human T cells, telomerase activity increases with acute antigen exposure but decreases with repeated antigen stimulation and as cells approach senescence.

The cellular environment also plays an important role in regulating telomere length and telomerase activity. At least in vitro, oxidative stress can shorten telomeres, while antioxidants and other natural elements can slow the shortening. A special oxidative damage to DNA has been proven in leukocytes in stressed women.

Given these observed links, the hypothesis that chronic psychological stress can lead to telomere shortening, and decreased telomerase function in peripheral blood mononuclear cells (PBMCs), is compelling.

Plausible explanation

The discovery of telomerases initially solved the problem of replicating the ends of linear DNA molecules, since this enzyme, a ribonucleoprotein, due to its activity, is essential for both the protein component and the RNA.

Telomerases differ from all polymerases in that they use an internal template rather than an external one, which imposes specific limitations on primer elongation and catalysis (increase in chemical reaction).

Telomerase elongates the starter DNA by adding one by one the triphosphate deoxynucleotides (monometers that constitute DNA) and thus generates telomere repeats.

The enzyme also has endonucleolytic activity (cuts in one or more strands of the double helix) that could be related to a correction function. It contains telomerase RNA with a sector complementary to the telomere sequence. The union of telomeric DNA with telomerase RNA occurs by complementary base pairing.

The enzyme lengthens the telomere using RNA as a template and upon completing one lengthening the enzyme moves and begins a new lengthening cycle and so on.

Changes from one amino acid to another produce telomere shortening and senescence in yeast, indicating their importance for telomere lengthening in vivo.

Telomerase and the aging process

The level of telomerase activity is important in determining telomere length in cells and tissues in aging.

The importance of telomerase reactivation is evaluated, both for the development of cancer and for the immortalization of cells for therapeutic processes.

Since telomeres are the specialized repetitive DNA sequences at the ends of linear chromosomes, and associated proteins, that serve to maintain the integrity of the chromosomes, telomerase, a ribonucleoprotein polymerase complex, maintains telomere length. In the absence of telomerase activity, telomeres progressively shorten.

Telomerase activity is absent in most normal human somatic cells due to lack of expression of TERT (telomerase reverse transcriptase) although TERC (RNA component of telomerase) is generally present. On the other hand, most mouse cells have telomerase activity, and without it telomere shortening eventually limits cell growth, either by senescence, in cells with intact cell cycle controls (cell cycle block). , or by crises in cells with inactivated checkpoints (telomere fusions cause chromosome breakage and mitotic catastrophe).

Expression of TERT in cells that otherwise lack telomerase activity causes the cells to avoid senescence and crisis, and such cells are commonly referred to as "immortalized."

The absence of telomerase activity in most human somatic cells results in telomere shortening during aging. Telomerase activity can be restored to human cells by transduction of the hTERT gene or potentially by medicinal plant therapy.

Does telomerase activity determine aging?

The first aspect of this question is whether differences in aging rates between mammalian species are caused in whole or in part by species-specific differences in telomerase/telomere biology.

A very brief examination of this question leaves us with a doubt as an answer. Mice are short-lived compared to humans, however, mice have long telomeres and adult mouse somatic cells often have telomerase activity.

Do you mean that it is the same in humans? As far as we know, humans have relatively short telomeres, even when compared to closely related primates, and telomerase activity is very low in most cells except some types of stem cells, in the germ line and some. somatic cells such as T lymphocytes.

If telomere attrition were a major cause of aging, one would expect humans to be relatively susceptible to this process and mice to be resistant. But in the same way that mice are extremely sensitive to increases in cholesterol, while humans can consume very high amounts for years, we must consider that the influence of telomeres is more decisive, in terms of longevity, in humans. than in mice. Or perhaps it is that the short lifespan of mice compared to that of humans does not allow time for telomere problems to manifest.

CHAPTER 6

STRESS

Accelerated telomere shortening in response to stress

Numerous studies demonstrate links between chronic stress and rates of poor health, including risk factors for cardiovascular disease and poor immune function. However, the exact mechanisms of how stress undermines health are dubious, essentially because stress is not an evil, but rather an adaptation mechanism.

The hypothesis is that stress affects health by modulating the rate of cellular aging. Oxidation, overload and cell apoptosis are the most plausible conclusions. We found evidence that psychological stress, both perceived stress and stress chronicity, are significantly associated with increased oxidative stress (the imbalance between free radicals and antioxidants), lower telomerase activity, and shorter telomere length. , known determinants of senescence and cellular longevity in peripheral blood mononuclear cells from healthy patients.

Premenopausal women, with the highest levels of perceived stress, have shorter telomeres on average, and a decade of additional aging, compared to women with low stress.

These findings have implications for understanding how, at the cellular level, stress can promote the early onset of age-related diseases.

People who are stressed for long periods tend to show dark circles under their eyes, and psychological stress is commonly thought to lead to premature aging and related diseases, including risk factors for cardiovascular disease and worse immune function. However, the exact mechanisms of how this stress exerts these effects are not well known, including whether stress accelerates aging at the cellular level and how cellular aging translates into aging of the organism.

Recent research points to the crucial role of telomeres and telomerase in cellular aging and potentially disease. We remember that when cells divide, the telomere does not reproduce completely due to the limitations of DNA polymerases in completing the replication of the ends of linear molecules, which leads to its shortening with each repetition.

When telomeres shorten sufficiently, the cell enters senescence and doubles its errors in mitosis. In people, telomeres shorten with age in all replicating somatic cells that have been examined, including fibroblasts and leukocytes. Thus, telomere length can serve as a biomarker of a cell's biological, not chronological, age or potential for cell division.

The role of telomerase in stress

Telomerase, a cellular enzyme, adds the necessary telomeric DNA to the ends of the telomere, although it also has direct protective functions. In human T cells, telomerase activity increases with acute antigen exposure but decreases with repeated antigen stimulation and as cells approach senescence. In people with dyskeratosis congenita, a genetic disease that decreases the ability to synthesize enough telomerase, telomeres shorten and they die prematurely from progressive bone marrow failure and vulnerability to infections.

The cellular environment also plays an important role in regulating telomere length and telomerase activity. At least in vitro, oxidative stress can shorten telomeres, and antioxidants and other natural elements can slow the shortening. A special oxidative damage to DNA has been proven in leukocytes in stressed women.

Given these observed links, the hypothesis that chronic psychological stress can lead to telomere shortening, and decreased telomerase function in peripheral blood mononuclear cells (PBMCs), is compelling.

Evaluative methods

To study objective (event-based) and subjective (perception-based) stress, 58 healthy premenopausal women who were biological mothers of a healthy child (19 "control mothers" and 39 "caregiver mothers") were examined.

The latter were predicted to have, on average, greater environmental exposure to stress. Women in both groups completed a standardized 10-question questionnaire to assess their level of perceived stress in the past month. This design allowed us to examine the importance of perceived stress and objective stress measures (caregiver status and chronicity of stress based on number of years since diagnosis). All analyzes were carried out controlling for age because we wanted to test telomere shortening caused by stress, independent of the chronological age of the women, although assuming that age was related to telomere length.

Each subject was 20–50 years old (mean = 38 ± 6.5 years) and had at least one biological child living with her. Subjects were free of any current or chronic illness. The use of oral contraceptives was similar in the caregiver and control groups. The obesity index was quantified by body mass index (BMI): weight (in kilograms) and height (in meters). Blood was drawn on an empty stomach on one morning during the first 7 days of the follicular phase of the menstrual cycle.

Mean telomere length and telomerase activity were quantitatively measured in PBMCs (peripheral blood mononuclear cells) that were stored frozen at -80°C. Telomere length values were measured from DNA using a quantitative PCR (polymerase chain reaction) assay that determines the relative relationship between the number of telomere repeat copies to the number of single-copy copies (ratio T/S), in experimental samples compared to a reference DNA sample. Telomerase activity was measured by the telomerase repeat amplification protocol with a commercial kit and all values used were in the linear quantitative range.

Vitamin E (alpha-tocopherol) was measured with HPLC (liquid chromatography) from serum isolated from a foil-protected blood sample.

The level of F2-isoprostanes, a reliable measure of oxidative stress, was quantified from a 12-hour nocturnal urine sample in 44 women (urine was not collected in the first 14 subjects) using a chromatography/mass spectrometry. and adjusting creatinine levels. An oxidative stress index was calculated with vitamin E that represents the effect of oxidative stress, taking into account antioxidant defenses.

Regarding women caring for young children, the average perceived stress level was significantly higher in caregivers than in controls. As a group, caregivers did not differ from controls in telomere length, telomerase activity, or oxidative stress index, but the duration of their chronic stress (number of years as a caregiver) varied greatly (from 1 to 12 years). In fact, within the group of caregivers, the more years of caregiving, the shorter the mother's telomere length, the lower the telomerase activity and the greater the oxidative stress.

We also found significant correlations between perceived stress and the three markers of cellular aging in the entire sample of caregivers and non-caregivers. In particular, telomere length was related to perceived stress in both caregivers and controls. Therefore, the relationship between perceived stress and shorter telomeres is not simply due to the severe stress experienced by many of the caregivers, but rather to continuity in stress levels.

Because telomere length decreases during normal aging, one can estimate the years of aging that are expected to pass to bring telomeres to a delicate state. Therefore, when we associate telomere shortening with years of aging, we base our estimates on studies that average telomere shortening across adulthood. Thus, the shortening in the high-stress group indicates that their lymphocytes had aged the equivalent of 9-17 additional years, compared to the low-stress group. Furthermore, the high stress group also had significantly lower telomerase activity and higher oxidative stress than the low stress group. Mean telomerase activity, adjusted for BMI and age, was 48% lower in the high stress group.

Discussion

The exact mechanisms that connect the mind to the cell are unknown, although it is well accepted that cellular senescence may include stress-induced processes. The current findings suggest that stress-induced premature senescence in people could be influenced by chronic or perceived life stress. It remains to study the benefits produced by pleasurable activities and the satisfaction of life. Maybe there should be more psychologists who listen to people's happiness, and not just their sorrows.

Psychological stress could affect cellular aging through at least three non-exclusive pathways: immune cell function or distribution, oxidative stress, or telomerase activity. It would also affect the neuroendocrine system, since there is a relationship between stress hormones and oxidative stress. Glucocorticoids, the primary adrenal hormones secreted during stress, increase oxidative stress damage in neurons, in part by increasing glutamate and calcium, and decreasing antioxidant enzymes.

It is also notable that, in women, distress has been linked to increased oxidative DNA damage. In this sense, it is important to point out the inconvenience of administering anxiolytics and tranquilizers in situations of stress, physical or mental, as this further nullifies the body's response to adapt to conflictive situations. The adaptogens offered by natural medicine are usually the best option. When adaptogens and natural energizers are administered, telomere length is restored and lifespan is prolonged.

It is unknown whether resistance to physiological stress is related to resistance to psychological stress, but it seems certain that this is the case.

By strengthening the body, making it resistant, the mind assumes the benefit.

These associations between stress and cellular aging have clinically significant implications for human health. A 50% deficiency in telomerase RNA gene dosage caused by dyskeratosis congenita is sufficient to cause premature death in adults due to bone marrow failure and vulnerability to infections. In the elderly, telomere shortening is strongly associated with higher mortality rates. Finally, patients with early myocardial infarction had leukocyte telomere lengths equivalent to those typical of a person 11 years older than controls, similar to the magnitude of accelerated cellular aging observed in the high-stress group.

In summary, psychological stress is associated with indicators of accelerated cellular aging: oxidative stress, telomere length and telomerase activity in PBMCs.

Many questions remain, such as whether shorter telomeres in leukocytes lead to earlier immunological senescence and relate to shorter telomeres in other proliferative cells, such as cardiovascular endothelium.

CHAPTER 7

GENES AND TELOMERES

The question of whether differences in telomere biology are important determinants of aging and lifespan among individuals within a species is only significant in species such as humans that have limited telomerase activity. What we also know is that mice with defects in the TERC gene suffer from telomere shortening and in later generation telomerase-deficient mice, various organs have altered functions, demonstrating that sufficiently short telomeres have an adverse impact on tissue function. . So experiments in mice cannot answer the question of whether telomeres ever reach a "critical" length, that is, a length that impairs proliferation (or possibly some other cellular property) in any tissue in humans over a lifetime. normal.

The few conclusive tests that have been performed in humans demonstrated that certain changes observed in older individuals, such as anemia and slow wound healing, a consequence of altered cell proliferation, were an anticipated consequence of shortened telomeres.

Despite the lack of clear evidence for impaired proliferation in aging, there is indeed good evidence for progressive telomere shortening in many human cell types, including peripheral white blood cells, smooth muscle cells, endothelial cells, epithelial cells. , and adrenocortical cells, among others. One example is of particular interest: proliferative capacity is closely related to telomere length in endothelial cells. Telomere lengths in endothelial cells decreased as a function of donor age, with a greater decrease observed in cells isolated from the iliac artery compared to cells from the thoracic artery.

The greatest decrease in telomere length was observed in cells that had likely undergone more proliferation in vivo, as they resided in a part of the vascular system where blood flow could cause more chronic damage to the endothelium.

Therefore, telomere shortening effectively occurs in the human body during aging. The question, as stated above, is whether this telomere shortening is a determinant of differences in aging and lifespan between individuals.

Two aspects of this question are:

>(1) Whether telomere length, measured in specific cell populations in the body, correlates with longevity or disease.

>(2) Whether telomere shortening in any cell population causes functional impairment of that population.

Currently the only cell populations that have been subjected to the required depth of analysis are peripheral white blood cells and some white blood cell subsets.

However, telomere analyzes now provide very significant data: people who have chronic diseases have shortened telomeres. People who enter into accelerated aging, too. Finally, centenarians typically have optimal telomere length.

Several observational studies have attempted to gain insight into the question of whether age-related telomere shortening in human peripheral white blood cells is associated with health and disease status. One study concluded that "by itself, socioeconomic status appears to have an impact on white blood cell telomere dynamics." Another study of mothers of children with chronic diseases concluded that "psychological stress is associated with indicators of accelerated cellular aging, including shorter telomere length." Both studies suggest an influence of perceived psychological state on telomere length. Of course, psychological stress does not necessarily cause stress at the cellular/molecular level if the individual adapts.

A plausible link is the endocrine system and possibly the explanation for the differences in telomere length in individuals of different psychological status is found in the actions of hormones such as glucocorticoids that cause cell death and malignant cell proliferation in the hematopoietic system.

However, and this must be very clear, glucocorticoids are essential hormones for life and when they increase due to stress they have a protective physiological function not against the course of the stress response, but as a safeguard, preventing them from being generated. exaggerated defense responses activated by stress.

When the protective response is continued and very high, it becomes detrimental in its attempt to maintain the threatened homeostasis.

Some clinical proceedings have addressed the question of whether short telomeres in peripheral white blood cells cause functional impairment. In bone marrow transplant recipients, the hematopoietic system can undergo dramatic telomere shortening, perhaps the equivalent of several decades of "aging." Some data suggest that long-term survivors of bone marrow transplants may suffer immune dysfunction as a consequence of the combination of sudden loss of telomere length at the time of transplantation, followed by normal age-related shortening.

This area of research, that is, the epidemiological correlations between white cell telomere length and longevity or disease, is a complex topic and needs a general review. One aspect should be mentioned, and that is that global changes in telomere length could be the result of changes in subsets of cells. This context is of interest, since the expansion of T lymphocytes is associated with mortality.

Other lymphocytes have shorter telomeres than other white blood cells from the same individual and this may be related to the observation that loss of CD28 expression is also associated with loss of ability of T lymphocytes to increase telomerase activity.

It must be remembered that no observational study, whether in the entire white blood cell population or in subsets, can establish cause and effect.

Such studies, therefore, of total white blood cells and T lymphocyte subsets, confirm that they can have excessive cell proliferation, as a result of various causes, which leads to telomere shortening. What is certain is that telomere shortening is associated with age, and that it causes aging and hair loss, as well as a senile appearance of the skin. These age-related changes are the result of profound alterations in melanocytes, including melanocyte stem cells.

There are at least three important questions that need to be answered:

> First, we need to know what telomere length in human tissues is associated with functional impairment, of specific organs, tissues or cell populations.
>
> Second, because of the large heterogeneity in telomere lengths between cells and between different telomeres within cells, we need to know whether there could be deterioration of individual

cells even if there is no measurable deficit in the cell population. as a whole.

And third, we don't know if telomere length in white blood cells, or T cells, correlates with telomere length in other tissues.

Access to appropriate tissue samples to test this is problematic, as is there a specific cell population in the body in which telomere length directly determines differences in health, disease or the actual rate of aging between humans? individual? This is possible, but we need more evidence.

Telomeres, telomerase and mutations

Another important question that is repeatedly raised in this review is whether high or low telomerase activity could be a factor causing a shorter or longer lifespan. In fact, it is speculated that short telomeres and a lack of telomerase may exert a longevity-promoting effect through cancer prevention. This is a mistake, since tumor cells are confused with healthy cells. Furthermore, not all fatal diseases are carcinogenic. As we have said, cancer cells produce and activate their own telomerase, which is why they survive; They do not depend on organic telomerase itself. Obviously, short telomeres or a lack of telomerase do not produce optimal aging, quite the contrary. The challenge is to deactivate telomerase only in tumor cells, sparing the healthy ones.

It is also reasonable to hypothesize that any species that has evolved a slower rate of aging will also need to develop mechanisms to reduce susceptibility to premature death from cancer. The short telomere and lack of telomerase combination act as a tumor suppressor mechanism in mammals, as detailed below.

Telomere shortening eventually leads to cellular senescence, a permanent form of growth arrest. It refers to the number of times normal cells can divide before senescence is a constant for a particular cell population, thus giving rise to the idea of a mitotic clock.

As far as we know, the processes of senescence and telomere shortening are closely linked and were often discussed as a single phenomenon. It later became clear that telomere shortening was just one of many ways in which cells could become senescent. If we do not rely on the telomere mechanism, senescence-induced oncogenes represent one of the two mechanisms by which senescence exerts an anticancer effect. The complex topic of oncogene-induced senescence has been reviewed numerous times, without clear conclusions.

The second mechanism studied refers to the fact that telomere shortening in a normal cell is not the most determining factor, but is probably the operation of telomere shortening in a progressively abnormal cell clone.

The reasoning for this statement is the following: if a cell clone is normal, without oncogenic activation, then by definition it reaches a state of critically short telomeres, at which point the cell stops dividing, but does not prevent cancer. If the oncogene is activated as well as its dependent DNA, senescence damage occurs, so a shortened telomere would not act to prevent cancer.

Furthermore, it is very likely that in cells in which multiple oncogenic mutations have occurred, the limitation of cell division imposed by shortened telomeres is a final way for the body to eliminate a potentially harmful clone from the cells. This is a terminal state for the clone, unless it escapes by becoming immortal. A cell clone that has avoided elimination by apoptosis, senescence, or differentiation over many cell generations has probably acquired multiple mutations. Most developed cancer cells have a large number of mutations and, for example, in human colorectal and breast cancers they have an average of ~90 mutant genes, of which a somewhat smaller number are required for the neoplastic properties of the cell.

To simplify: telomere shortening causes disease, accelerated aging, and eventually death. Weakening or preventing the optimal maintenance of telomeres is a serious mistake, as would not feeding the patient to try to kill the malignant cells.

When faced with an illness, the body must have an adequate level of energy to withstand that illness, this energy level being more important than the illness itself. It is as if we were trying to improve a forest by acting on a few tree species, rather than as a whole.

Anticancer mechanisms

Senescence can be triggered by an oncogenic mutation, a protein that stimulates cell proliferation and triggers senescence. Because such cells have undergone extreme telomere shortening, they reach a state called "crisis." In this state, short dysfunctional telomeres cause end-to-end chromosome fusions, leading to increasing aneuploidy (changes in chromosome number), mitotic catastrophe, a failure of cytokinesis, multipolar cell division, and macroscopic aberrations in the number of chromosomes.

Mitotic catastrophe leads to the arrest of mitosis, or the formation of cells with multiple nuclei or a single giant nucleus, something often seen in human cancers.

An obvious question is why telomerase-negative cancers that have a history of self-limiting growth are not seen clinically, perhaps because some cancers grow widely and then stop due to a lack of telomerase. Cancers that lack telomerase and do not acquire sufficient telomerase activity probably never grow large enough to be clinically detectable.

The exception to this statement may be dermatological cancers, which are more likely to be detected in very early stages. Small squamous cell carcinomas may lack a telomere maintenance mechanism. In a human being, a cancer may be clinically undetectable, and after the cells go into crisis they die, leaving little trace of the existence of the neoplasm.

There are cells from experimental tumors that go into crisis and do not die by apoptosis, but ultimately die through nonspecific necrosis that occurs after the tumor stops enlarging. As early cancer detection improves, it may be more common to find very small malignant lesions that lack telomere maintenance mechanisms.

If at some point during the growth of the clone or in the crisis, the cells within the clone acquire a sufficient level of telomerase activity for telomere maintenance, then the crisis can be avoided. Most cancer cells have activated telomere maintenance mechanisms, mainly as a result of increased expression of TERT. Therefore, the lack of telomerase, or the lack of sufficient telomerase activity to allow immortal growth, exerts a significant barrier to the formation of a lethal cancer from a clone of cells that otherwise has a set of mutations that render it They give carcinogenic properties.

In human cells the combination of short telomeres in tumor cells and suppression of TERT expression together provide an anti-cancer mechanism.

The existence of this anticancer mechanism may be a factor that contributes to the great difference in susceptibility to cancer. However, and I must insist on this, the same combination of short telomeres and the lack of TERT expression in healthy cells could limit the ability of tissues to respond to stress and old age.

The potential role of telomerase in cell therapy

From the first reports of immortalization, it was speculated that the technology could be used to expand cell populations to later make a therapeutic transplant. This was considered particularly important for the replacement of tissues and organs damaged during aging. In this therapy, cells with shortened telomeres would be isolated from a patient and telomere length would be restored by expression of hTERT (telomerase reverse transcriptase). The cell population would be expanded in culture and then the cells would be reintroduced into the body to restore tissue and organ function. These cells would have specific properties, like stem cells or genetically modified cells.

The combination of immortalization and alteration of gene expression could make hTERT-immortalized cells particularly attractive for cell therapy and related technologies such as tissue engineering. A variety of hTERT-modified cells have been used in experimental cell therapy and a recent example is the construction of engineered blood vessels with hTERT-expressing smooth muscle cells.

hTERT does not cooperate with known oncoproteins in tumorigenesis and only when telomeres have shortened to a critical level is telomerase activity necessary for continued tumor growth. The question to consider is whether this modification of hTERT could make cells more dangerous in vivo.

Fortunately, in all the experiments that have been performed using bovine and human adrenocortical cells, as well as human fibroblasts, sporadic tumor formation from hTERT-modified cells was never observed.

The ability of hTERT to exert a variety of effects that counteract cell death is surprising and these effects have also been demonstrated in animals. In mice this protects against heart failure and has many other effects on the cardiovascular system and chromosomal damage caused by ionizing radiation. Changes in gene expression in the hTERT-modified cells allow them to survive and grow in sites in the body where they would not otherwise grow, such as the subcutaneous space, which is essentially a tough place for even the most robust cells to survive.

Conclusions

Telomere shortening resulting from the absence of telomerase activity may be a factor in determining some age-related properties of organs in humans.

Telomerase reactivation could be useful in some forms of cell therapy and does not appear to present a safety concern. However, telomerase activation removes a barrier to the continued growth of developing cancers, as the lack of telomerase activity provides a tumor suppressor function. As we have said, the key is that cancer cells activate their own telomerase.

CHAPTER 8

EPIGENETICS

Genes give us the potential, but they do not determine the outcome. It all depends on the environment that decides the final result.

What is Epigenetics?

Epigenetics is the study of potentially heritable changes in gene expression (active versus inactive genes) that do not involve changes in the underlying DNA sequence - a change in phenotype without a change in genotype - which, in turn, affects , to how cells read genes.

The term "epigenetics" was first used to refer to the complex interactions between the genome and the environment that are involved in development and differentiation in higher organisms. Currently, this term is used to refer to hereditary disorders that are not due to changes in the DNA sequence. Rather, epigenetic modifications or "tags," such as DNA methylation and histone modification, alter DNA accessibility and chromatin structure, thereby regulating gene expression patterns.

These processes are crucial for the normal development and differentiation of different cell lineages in the adult organism and can be modified by exogenous influences and, as such, can contribute to or be the result of environmental alterations of the phenotype or pathophenotype, understanding as such the endotypes with which people are grouped based on the hormonal design that dominates their metabolism.

In 2006, for example, more than 2,500 articles related to epigenetics were published and in 2010, more than 13,000, reaching 17,000 in 2013. However, this number is now surpassed, with epigenetic concepts extending to fields such as ecology. and psychology. Alternative medicines, on the other hand, want to insist that by modifying our environment and using exclusively natural elements, we can silence or activate inherited behaviors and characteristics. The problem is that, until now, the subject "epigenetics" is not included in medical curricula.

The lack of a clear definition has led to confusion and misuse of the term, while also making research within the field of epigenetics difficult to synthesize and reconcile. We should also expand the field of study of epigenetics to branches such as chemistry, physics, ecology and even psychology, not exclusively delegating the experiments and conclusions to biology. And, as usual, we will provide the suggestions provided by Natural Medicine -until now largely excluded- in the solution of health problems through epigenetics.

History

To understand the meaning of the term epigenetics, we must understand the context in which it was derived. Conrad Waddington, who first defined the field in 1942, worked as an embryologist and developmental biologist. In 1947, he founded and headed the first department of genetics at the Edinburgh Institute and later formed his own research group.

Waddington had a great appreciation for genetics and was a leading advocate of uniting genetic principles with other fields of biology, such as cytology, embryology, and evolutionary biology; However, he was particularly interested in embryology and developmental genetics, specifically the mechanisms that controlled cellular differentiation. At the time, there were two prevailing views on development, both derived from the 17th century: preformation, which claimed that all adult characteristics were already present in the embryo and simply needed to grow or unfold, and epigenesis, which postulated that The new tissues were created from successive interactions between the constituents of the embryo. It seems that the latter conclusion was the prevailing one, but Waddington believed that both preformation and epigenesis could be complementary, with preform representing the static nature of the gene and epigenesis representing the dynamic nature of gene expression. That is why through the combination of these concepts he coined the term epigenetics, which he referred to as "the branch of biology that studies the causal interactions between genes and their products that lead the phenotype to be."

It is important to note that genetics was still a young field at the time, centered on Mendel's work on the inheritance of traits, with the gene being accepted as the unit of heredity; but little was known about the biochemical nature of the gene or how it worked. It was not until

Beadle and Tatum, in 1941, published their work affirming the concept of gene and enzyme, that the understanding of gene function took discrete shape and subsequent work in molecular biology defined gene structure. This genocentric atmosphere, along with the emerging effort to understand gene regulation and expression, had a strong influence on the creation of epigenetics, both as a concept and as a field of study, something that did not arrive until 2002.

At that time, many were interested in the process of gene control and expression. Certain experimental embryologists and geneticists studied mutations by inducing changes in development through experimentation with chemicals. Waddington (died 1975), on the other hand, was more interested in the cellular processes that caused these changes, than in the stimuli that created them.

One of his most important contributions was his recognition and emphasis on the flexible relationship between genotype and phenotype, and this was an idea that many of his contemporaries took up. Today, Waddington's views on epigenetics are more closely associated with phenotypic plasticity, which is the ability of a gene to produce multiple effects. But he also coined the term canalization to refer to the inherent stability of certain phenotypes (developmental traits) across different genotypes and environments.

In 1958, 16 years after Waddington coined the term, David Nanney published a paper in which he used the term epigenetics to distinguish between different types of cellular control systems. He proposed that genetic components were responsible for maintaining and perpetuating a library of genes, expressed and unexpressed, through a template replication mechanism. He then considered epigenetic components as auxiliary mechanisms that controlled the expression of specific genes. Most importantly, in addition to discussing variability in expression patterns, Nanney emphasized the fact that expression states could persist through cell division. Although some consider that Nanney used the term epigenetic, while Waddington spoke of paragenetics, the overlap is considerable. It is clear, however, that Nanney's contemplation of the stability of cellular expression states was an important addition to

Waddington's ideas, which had significant impacts on the future direction of epigenetics.

Definitions of Epigenetics

As we see, while Waddington was more interested in genetic regulation and genotype-phenotype interactions, Nanney and Lederberg were more interested in the stability of cellular expression and inheritance states. Even today, this has led to a certain identity crisis in definition.

Throughout the 1980s and 1990s, the definition of epigenetics moved away from developmental processes and became more generalized. For example, a 1982 definition describes epigenetics as "pertaining to the interaction of genetic factors and the developmental processes through which the genotype is expressed in the phenotype (Lincoln). This definition includes the term development, but its meaning It appears to relate more to the development of phenotype than to an ontological meaning. Although only slightly different from Waddington's original definition, this definition and others during this time expanded the meaning of epigenetics significantly and made it more available and applicable to others. fields, emphasizing the importance of genetic and non-genetic factors in controlling gene expression, while downplaying the connection with development.

In the 1970s and 1980s, experiments on the relationship between DNA methylation, cell differentiation and gene expression became more closely associated with epigenetics. Work on cellular memory and DNA methylation, particularly the finding that DNA methylation had strong effects on gene expression and that these effects persisted through mitosis, was welcomed. That is why epigenetics was redefined in a more specific *way and focused on the inheritance of expression states* (and not epigenetic inheritance, in which it did not include a specific component on heritability). Some proposed two different definitions, insufficient when used separately, but covering all currently recognized epigenetic processes when taken together. The first definition stated that epigenetics was "the study of changes in gene expression, which occur in organisms with differentiated cells, and the mitotic inheritance of certain gene expression patterns."

The second indicated that epigenetics was "nuclear inheritance, which is not based on differences in DNA sequence." Other researchers referred to the "study of changes in gene function that are heritable and do not involve change in DNA sequence."

The addition of heritability to Waddington's original definition was a significant change because, although it does not exclude the inheritance of expression states, this aspect was not a fundamental part of the concept of epigenetics. It was precisely the inability to explain these phenomena through simple genetic explanations that became a defining element of epigenetics. Before understanding RNA-based regulatory mechanisms, and still in the early stages of DNA methylation and histone modifications, the uncoupling of genotype and phenotype, well defined by epigenetics, managed to perfectly describe the disconnection between a gene and their phenotype, already avoiding metaphors. This included occasions in which the expression of a gene varied depending on its location, its imprinting (a genetic phenomenon by which certain genes are expressed in a specific way that depends on the sex of the parent), or other circumstances, for example, the establishment of centromeres and restoration of telomeres. The "new genetics" had been born.

It is not difficult to find articles in current scientific literature that use the term epigenetics to explain previous definitions, or other new ones, but it is necessary to clarify so that we do not encounter a problem similar to the concept of metaphysics. And what's worse, a dichotomy within the field of epigenetics.

Waddington's epigenetics describes the interaction of genetic and cytoplasmic elements that produce emergent phenotypes and those that in the biological sciences are explained as interactions between the gene and the environment, between the expression of phenotypes mediated by the environment, particularly in the fields of The ecology.

Those that are related to DNA methylation, chromatin activity states, chromosomal imprinting, centromeric function, etc. There is great interest in knowing how expression patterns persist across different cells (mitosis) and generations (meiosis). Although the underlying mechanisms are very different, they all use the same term: epigenetics.

This apparent ambiguity has made the task of identifying epigenetic phenomena difficult and also limits more advanced efforts to determine how epigenetic processes occur. It seems that semantics are making investigations difficult. To us it seems simple to understand and define, but we see that many scientists are more concerned about where to place what they are researching or that their name appears in some way in history.

It seems that the biggest problem is knowing whether Waddington's epigenetics is the same or complementary to Holliday's epigenetics, although some believe that they are not necessarily related to each other.

Perhaps the economic movements that are being related to this are to blame, and the geneticists and medical laboratories dedicated to traditional genetics are not interested in rectifying their, until now, supported conclusions.

The second challenge is to address the methodological problems that have accumulated within the field of epigenetics over time, due to the absence of a clear definition. Rather than building from clear first principles, the field of epigenetics remains a trap to baffle new scholars and prevent them from disqualifying the categorizations and justifications that were previously developed. Working backwards to reevaluate the first principles of epigenetics will help put the field on a stronger track and hopefully allow research to flourish.

So Bird, in 2007, proposed that epigenetics could be redefined as "the structural adaptation of chromosomal regions to record, signal, or perpetuate altered states of activity." Later, in 2014, he offered the term "memigenetics" to denote states of expression that are heritable. Perhaps we could redefine epigenetics as "the study of the phenomena and mechanisms that cause linked chromosomes, and heritable changes to gene expression that do not depend on changes in DNA sequence." This definition does not exclude a priori any unit of inheritance, including protein-coding genes, telomeres, centromeres, functional RNA gene products, origins of replication, genome instabilities, or anything else that may manifest a phenotype.

The concept of hereditary memory (more than "inheritance") is also included, and in development the influence of stress on the pregnant mother and her offspring is discussed for the first time.

These genetic factors, which are determined by the cellular environment rather than by heredity, intervene in the determination of ontogeny (development of an organism, from fertilization of the zygote in sexual reproduction to its senescence, passing through the adult form) and which also intervenes in the heritable regulation of genetic expression without change in the nucleotide sequence. It can be said –simplifying– that epigenetics is the set of chemical reactions and other processes that modify the activity of DNA, but without altering its sequence.

Epigenetic modifications can commonly manifest, such as when cells differentiate to become skin cells, liver cells, brain cells, etc. Sometimes these changes can have detrimental effects, resulting in diseases such as cancer.

Gene silencing, caused by modifications in DNA and RNA, can initiate and maintain epigenetic change. So important are these changes that many human disorders and fatal diseases can be due to this. Sometimes genes are activated, giving rise to latent diseases. However, predictive medicine, which "predicts" the diseases that are going to develop – within a framework of probabilities – ignores possible genetic modifications caused by the individual's environment. As a pernicious example, is the damage they caused to actress Angelina Jolie to allow her to have a double mastectomy and subsequently the removal of her ovaries.

More suggestive –and plausible– is the possibility of restoring telomere shortening related to tumor growth and disruptive changes in gene expression. Using positive thinking or mindfulness exercises, some researchers found that those who participated in these therapies maintained their telomere length.

It is not the only therapeutic resource, but it seems adequate. The epigenetic influence was demonstrated.

Evolution to current epigenetics

What began as extensive research focused on the combination of genetics and biology by highly respected scientists, including the aforementioned Conrad H. Waddington and Ernst Hadorn, in the mid-20th century, has evolved into the field that is today referred to as epigenetics. The initial term epigenetics described the influence of genetic processes on development. During the 1990s there was renewed interest in genetic assimilation and this led to the observation that environmental stress caused the genetic assimilation of certain phenotypic characteristics. Since then, research efforts have focused on unraveling the epigenetic mechanisms related to these types of changes.

Currently, DNA methylation (an epigenetic mechanism used by cells to control gene expression) is one of the most widely studied and well-characterized epigenetic modifications dating back to studies by Griffith and Mahler in 1969, which suggested that methylation DNA may be important in long-term memory function. Other important modifications include chromatin

(DNA-protein complex within the nucleus of mammalian cells) remodeling, histone modifications (basic proteins that bind to DNA), and non-coding RNA pathways.

This noncoding RNA, made up of small pieces, can bind to specific RNA molecules and prevent cells from using RNA to make a protein or function in other ways. Non-coding RNA, which can be used to block the production of proteins that the cell needs to grow, is associated with gene silencing and is currently considered an element to initiate and maintain epigenetic change.

Another source of study is the relationship between epigenetic changes and a series of diseases including various types of cancer, mental, immunological, neuropsychiatric and pediatric disorders. Since it is a regular and natural occurrence, it can also be influenced by various factors, including age, environment, lifestyle and disease status. Epigenetic modifications can manifest as commonly as the way cells terminally differentiate into different cells. Or, epigenetic change can have more detrimental effects that can result in diseases such as cancer.

Additionally, we can say that:

Epigenetics controls genes and certain circumstances in life can cause genes to be silenced or expressed over time. In other words, they can be off (become dormant) or on (be active).

Epigenetics is all around us. What we eat, where we live, who we interact with, when and where we sleep, how we move, even aging, all of these can eventually cause chemical modifications around genes that will turn them on or off over time. Furthermore, in certain diseases such as cancer or Alzheimer's, several genes will be modified, far from the normal and healthy state.

Epigenetics determines who we are now. Even though we are all human, why do some of us have blonde hair or darker skin? Well, this seems to be a genetic thing. But why do some of us hate the taste of mushrooms or eggplants? Why are some of us more sociable than others? Why do we change over time and what we liked before now bores us? The social and family world knows a lot about this.

The different combinations of genes that are turned on or off is what makes each of us unique. Furthermore, there are indications that some epigenetic changes may be acquired as a result of the immediate environment or perhaps also the distant one?

With over 20,000 genes, is it possible to predict the outcome of different combinations of genes being turned on or off? Maybe not for the human mind, but think about the computers of now and those of the future.

It will be as easy as when a vulgar calculator gives us the answer in seconds. The possible arrangements are enormous.

When we can correlate each cause and effect of the different combinations, and if we could reverse the state of the gene to maintain the good by eliminating the bad, then we could theoretically cure cancer, slow aging, stop obesity and perhaps even be happy.

Epigenetics and the environment

Our lifestyle is already influencing the new generations that accompany us and we are leaving a decisive mark on those not yet born. We are already writing their biography, their abilities and fears.

Fortunately, the study of epigenetics is growing rapidly and with it the understanding that both the environment and individual lifestyle can also interact directly with the genome to influence epigenetic change. These changes can be reflected at various stages of a person's life and even in later generations. For example, human epidemiological studies have provided evidence that prenatal and early postnatal environmental factors influence the adult risk of developing several chronic diseases and behavioral disorders. We would no longer talk about genetic or even congenital diseases, but epigenetic diseases, absolutely controllable. Studies have shown that children born during the Dutch famine period of 1944-1945 had increased rates of coronary heart disease and obesity after maternal exposure to the famine during early pregnancy, compared with those not exposed to the famine. famine. DNA methylation of the insulin-like growth factor II (IGF2) gene, a well-characterized epigenetic locus (marker), was found to be associated with this exposure. Likewise, it has been shown that adults who were prenatally exposed to starvation conditions have a significantly higher incidence of schizophrenia.

Importantly, epigenetic programming plays a crucial role in regulating pluripotency genes, which become inactive during differentiation. Since all organs contain more than one type of cell, the most suitable cell in regenerative therapy would be a stem cell that: 1) has a high capacity for self-renewal and regenerative potential and 2) is capable of generating tissues with cells from the three layers. germ cells (for example, parenchyma, connective tissue, vessels, nervous tissue, etc.). Cells that meet these requirements would be pluripotent cells.

Here, we review the main mechanisms in epigenetic regulation, with the role of long-term stable epigenetic modifications involving DNA methylation being notable. It is important to understand the role of nutritional and environmental challenges in generational inheritance and epigenetic modifications, focusing on examples that relate to complex cardiovascular diseases, especially the mechanisms by which homocysteine modifies epigenetic marks.

We remember that homocysteine is a sulfur amino acid important in the transfer of methyl groups in cellular metabolism, and that it is considered an influential factor in the development of cardiovascular and cerebrovascular diseases. Also, and most importantly, we will look at the possibilities of modifying therapeutically acquired epigenetic tags, analyzing currently available elements and speculating on future directions.

DNA sequence and heritability

Understanding why some genes are turned on or off is certainly less mysterious since the field of epigenetics was born, largely due to the identification of regulatory genes and gene-protein interactions. These findings explain much of the changes in Waddington gene expression, although difficulty remains in the consequences of heritability, the regulatory components that are encoded by DNA. However, epigenetics requires that the state of gene expression, not just the components necessary for gene expression, be heritable and not dependent on DNA sequence. We will explain some confusing concepts:

The term *dependency* refers to any molecule that cannot exist in the absence of DNA. However, the ability of the same DNA sequence to produce different expression profiles without a base pair change shows a lack of dependence on the primary sequence because something outside the sequence must be controlling expression.

A DNA *sequence* could refer to the euchromatic regions that contain the sequences that make up genes and encode proteins, and that are responsible for producing most of the proteins vital for cellular survival and function. Repetitive sequences, such as those present in heterochromatin, have been termed junk DNA. And if it's garbage, why study it? But it is likely that their function is poorly understood, and that the tools to investigate them are not developed. Recently, evidence has emerged that aspects of DNA other than the sequence of base pairs within genic regions are important for gene expression. Maybe we should redefine what a gene is.

Something very important, often overlooked, about DNA sequence is *localization*, which can affect gene expression in both coding and non-coding regions. So moving a gene sequence to a different location within the genome can affect its expression and that's where epigenetics comes in.

But the most conflictive term is *heritability*, since it has complicated defining what epigenetics is and its subsequent study. And time is as important as the beginning of something, and the prolonged or fleeting stimulus determines the changes.

Expressive changes cannot be required to persist through mitosis and/or meiosis for a phenotype to be considered epigenetic.

When something is heritable, it can also refer to the transfer of non-DNA molecules, whether methyl groups, histones, or cytoplasmic compounds. This occurs because inheritance is confused with transfer of molecules and it seems to be difficult to discern between changes in gene expression due to the inheritance of an expression state and those due to a real-time reaction to a stimulus. An example is when a parent cell or organism experiences a stimulus that causes a specific expression pattern and then a similar expression pattern is also evident in the offspring, without the offspring having experienced the initial stimulus.

If the germ cells respond to a stimulus experienced by the parent, there is no barrier between the stimulus and the offspring because the expression in the primordial cells of the future offspring is also directly affected.

Any stimulus that impacts a pregnant woman can affect the mother, the fetus, and the fetus's germ cells, including two additional generations of potential children. This implies that a similarity of expression would have to be shown between the mother and her great-granddaughter to verify a possible epigenetic connection. Therefore, if the expression pattern of the original germ cell were evident in the offspring, it is because there would be persistence through mitosis.

The main difficulty lies in identifying the mechanism of inheritance. If it is true that the compounds responsible for perpetuating an expression pattern have to be closely associated with DNA, as in methylation and chromatin modification, it would be necessary to consider that the transfer of cytoplasmic compounds really produces an effect on gene expression .

DNA methylation

DNA methylation is an epigenetic mechanism that occurs by adding a methyl group (CH_3) to DNA, often modifying gene function. These methyl groups project into the major groove of DNA and inhibit transcription.

Equally important in DNA demethylation, in the removal of a methyl group. This process is necessary for epigenetic reprogramming of genes and is also directly involved in many important disease mechanisms, such as tumor progression. As we have explained, this demethylation can be passive or active, or a combination of both.

Due to its heritability, DNA methylation is a powerful means of suppressing the expression of unwanted or excessive genes. Given the random nature of X chromosome inactivation, female carriers can show wide variation in the phenotypic expression of X-linked disorders.

A new mechanism involving specific DNA demethylation in response to hormonal stimulation has recently been discovered.

Transcriptional suppression by regulators can be alleviated by parathyroid hormone (PTH)-induced demethylation of CpG promoters.

This hormone-induced mechanism contrasts with repair and excision mechanisms, as it is directed to a specific promoter by hormonal action and does not require deamination. Although more studies are needed to confirm these mechanisms, the concept of hormone-induced methylation switching adds a new twist to epigenetic regulation.

Homocysteine and methylation reactions

Other methylation modifiers may also influence epigenetic tags. For example, dietary choline status (a betaine precursor involved in folate-independent pathways in methionine synthesis) was shown to affect DNA methylation. Additionally, betaine supplementation was shown in one study to attenuate atherosclerotic lesion formation and growth.

The regulation of vascular nitric oxide production can influence both atherogenesis and thrombosis. In this sense, and since nitric oxide is considered a molecule that modulates vascular tone that is produced during the conversion of L-arginine to L-citrulline, we must consider its essential role in smooth muscle relaxation, neurotransmission and immune cellular cytotoxicity.

Homocysteine is biochemically linked to the major epigenetic mark found in DNA.

Although increased circulating levels of homocysteine are a risk factor for vascular disease, recent clinical trials using folate and/or other vitamin B therapies to reduce it have failed to reduce rates of cardiovascular events, so they doubt on the direct causative role of homocysteine in vascular disease.

There are many in vivo examples suggesting that homocysteine (Hcy) levels can modulate global DNA methylation and several studies support the concept that DNA hypomethylation may be responsible, in part, for the vascular complications associated with increased circulating levels of Hcy. In patients with functional renal failure (and impaired homocysteine elimination), the risk of vascular disease increases.

Aberrant global DNA methylation is only one index of the potential for epigenetic dysregulation. Important are the rate of cell growth and DNA replication, chromatin accessibility, local availability of AdoMet (S-adenosyl methionine), nutritional factors including folate supplementation, duration and degree of the hyperhomocysteine state, inflammatory processes, dyslipidemias, oxidative stress and aging.

CHAPTER 9

EPIGENETICAL DAMAGES

By electromagnetic fields (EMFS) and extremely low frequencies (ELF)

The energy of electromagnetic waves is contained within packets of indivisible "quanta" that have to be radiated or absorbed as a whole.

Electrical Sensitivity (ES), Electromagnetic Sensitivity, EMF Sensitivity, Electrosensitivity, Electromagnetic Hypersensitivity (EHS), Electromagnetic Field Intolerance, Electrical Hypersensitivity, Microwave Sickness, Radiation Sickness, Radio Wave Sickness... many different terms that are used to describe this condition. The global term will be electromagnetic sensitivity.

Professor Olle Johansson of Sweden, one of the leading scientists working in this area, defines electrical sensitivity as a functional impairment that means different things to different people.

As societies industrialize and the technological revolution continues, there has been an unprecedented increase in the number and diversity of electromagnetic fields (EMFs). These sources include video display units (VDUs) associated with computers, mobile phones and their base stations. Although these devices have made our lives richer, safer and easier, they have been accompanied by concerns about possible health risks due to electromagnetic emissions.

There is no widely accepted definition and the World Health Organization (WHO) states on this topic: "EHS is characterized by a variety of non-specific symptoms, affecting individuals and attributed to exposure to electromagnetic fields. " The statement "attributed to exposure to electromagnetic fields" also attests to the controversy surrounding this issue. The WHO recognizes that these symptoms exist but does not attribute them, at least officially, to exposure to electromagnetic fields, something that for affected people is totally outrageous. Research into the health effects of exposure to these fields began in earnest in the 1960s and continues to this day. There is currently a huge amount of evidence proving the adverse health effects of electromagnetic fields, but public and even academic awareness remains very poor.

For some time now, a large number of people have reported a wide variety of health problems that are related to exposure to EMF (Electromagnetic Fields). While some people talk about mild symptoms and react by avoiding the fields as best they can, the others are so severely affected that they have had to quit work and change to another lifestyle.

This sensitivity has created a bad reputation towards EMF electromagnetic radiation, which is called "electromagnetic hypersensitivity" or EHS.

Static magnetic fields

There are few studies on the effects of static electric fields. According to the results obtained so far, the only acute effects are associated with movement of skin hair and discomfort caused by spark discharge. There is no effective research on the chronic or delayed effects of static electric fields, and it is believed that acute effects are only likely to occur when there is movement in the field, such as movement of a person, or internal body movement, such as movement. blood flow or heartbeat. A person moving in a field of more than 2 T (T=magnetic induction) may have sensations of vertigo and nausea, accompanied in some cases by a metallic taste in the mouth and perceptions of light flashes. Although they are only temporary, these effects can affect the safety of people carrying out sensitive operations.

Static magnetic fields influence electrical charges that move with the blood, such as ions, and generate electric currents and fields around the heart and large blood vessels, which can slightly alter blood circulation. Possible effects include slight disturbances in heartbeat and an increased risk of abnormal heart rhythms (arrhythmias), which can be life-threatening (such as ventricular fibrillation).

However, these acute effects only tend to occur with exposure to fields greater than 8 T.

To date, it has not been possible to determine whether there are long-term health consequences even in the case of exposure to fields whose intensity is measured in milliteslas, because adequate, long-term epidemiological studies with animals have not been carried out. For example, it is not possible to classify the carcinogenicity of static magnetic fields to humans. The lack of medical preparation is the cause of the delay in these studies.

The most commonly experienced symptoms include dermatological symptoms (redness, tingling and burning sensations), as well as neurasthenia and vegetative symptoms (fatigue, tiredness, concentration difficulties, dizziness, nausea, heart palpitations and digestive disorders). The set of symptoms is not part of any other recognized syndrome, so the cause-effect relationship is proven.

EHS resembles multiple chemical sensitivity (MCS), another disorder associated with low-level environmental exposures to chemicals. Electrically sensitive people react to computers, television, radio and music equipment, fluorescent lights, telephones, electronic security systems, power tools, electric sewing machines, electric heaters, and electric trains.

Electromagnetically sensitive people are typically sensitive to perfumes, pesticides, solvents, fluid cleaners, petrochemicals, diesel and formaldehyde. They also react to airborne particles and certain foods.

Both EHS and MCS are characterized by a series of nonspecific symptoms that lack apparent toxicological or physiological basis or independent verification.

A more general term for sensitivity to environmental factors is Idiopathic Environmental Intolerance (IEI), which originated from a workshop convened by the WHO International Program on Chemical Safety (IPCS) in 1996, in Berlin.

IEI is a descriptor without any implication of chemical etiology, immunological sensitivity or EMF susceptibility, which incorporates a number of disorders that share medically unexplained, non-specific, similar symptoms and that negatively affect people. However, the term EHS is in common use and continues to be used.

Studies on people with EHS

Certain studies have been conducted on people with EHS who were exposed to electromagnetic fields similar to those attributed to the cause of their symptoms. The goal was to provoke symptoms under controlled laboratory conditions.

Most studies indicate that people with EHS cannot detect exposure to EMF (Electromagnetic Fields) more accurately than non-EHS.

Double-blind controlled studies have always given controversial results.

It has been suggested that the symptoms experienced by some people with EHS may arise from environmental factors unrelated to EMF (Electromagnetic Radiation). Examples may include "flickering" of fluorescent lights, glare and other visual problems with computer screens, and poor ergonomic design of workstations. Other factors that may play a role include poor indoor air quality or stress in the workplace or living conditions.

Doctors sometimes claim that there is some indication that these symptoms may be due to pre-existing psychiatric conditions, as well as stress reactions resulting from concern about the health effects of EMF, rather than exposure. to EMF itself.

The patient, always according to his erroneous criteria, would be convinced of the origin of his illness, perhaps having read alarmist news, especially from those who sell tools to "eliminate" the electromagnetic fields that surround us.

However, it is enough for us to remember the unfortunate use of mercury alloy amalgams placed in the mouths of millions of patients, apparently harmless, to realize how some scientists minimize the severe damage caused by polluting agents. Once it is proven, everyone apologizes.

And we cannot forget the freon gas in refrigerators, asbestos and non-stick Teflon, once innocuous elements that time, and the dead, demonstrated to be poisons for human beings, although at the time they were considered by "scientists" , as harmless.

Data

Evidence of neurological effects of RFR

The neurological effects of RFR (Radio Frequency Radiation), published between 2007 and mid-2012, are outlined. Of these, 98 (63%) showed effects and 57 (37%) showed no effects.

Evidence for childhood leukemia:

Except for ionizing radiation, no other environmental factor has been so firmly established as a risk factor in childhood leukemia.

If so, the insistence on the primary involvement of the immune system would be confirmed.

There is sufficient evidence from epidemiological studies of an increased risk of exposure to power frequency magnetic fields (EMF) that cannot be attributed to chance, bias, or confounding factors.

Therefore, according to IARC (International Agency for Research on Cancer) rules, these exposures can be classified as a Group 1 carcinogen (known carcinogen).

Melatonin

The 13 published residential and occupational epidemiological studies consider that high ELF MF (Extremely Low Frequency Magnetic Fields) exposure can result in a decrease in melatonin. New research indicates that ELF MF exposure, in vitro, can significantly decrease melatonin activity through effects on MT1, an important melatonin receptor.

Although not affecting survival per se, prolonged ELF MF exposure alters the morphology of proliferating and differentiated cells, and significantly impairs antioxidant homeostasis and thiol content, triggering an increase in protein carbonylation.

Alzheimer's disease (AD)

There is now evidence that high levels of peripheral beta amyloid are a risk factor for AD and that high exposure to magnetic fields (MF) may increase peripheral beta amyloid.

DNA and stress

Stress proteins and DNA act as a fractal antenna for RFR. The spiral structure of the DNA coil in the core causes the molecule to react like a fractal antenna to a wide range of DNA, making them particularly vulnerable to EMF damage. The mechanism involves the direct interaction of electromagnetic fields (EMF) with the DNA molecule.

The activated cell stress response is a mechanism for cells exposed to a wide range of EMF frequencies to stimulate stress proteins (indicating an assault on the cell). Drs Lai and Singh discovered strand breaks in DNA exposed to radiofrequency radiation within levels considered "safe" in the US, UK and Canada.

The problem is that life on Earth did not evolve with biological protections or adaptive biological responses to these EMF radiation exposures. The human body is not prepared for it.

Heating

EMFs damage cells less than conventional electric heating.

Mother cells

Human stem cells are not adapted to chronic non-thermal microwave exposures (damaged DNA cannot be repaired), and DNA damage to genes in other cells is generally not repaired efficiently. The non-thermal effects of microwaves depend on various biological and physical parameters that must be taken into account when establishing safety standards.

New evidence suggests that the SAR (Specific Absorption Rate) concept, that is, the level of radiation exposure of a terminal, which has been widely adopted by safety standards, is not useful for the evaluation of risks to the health of non-thermal microwaves of mobile communication.

Other exposure parameters, such as frequency, modulation, duration and dose, must be taken into account.

Resonant frequencies can cause biological effects at very low intensities comparable to base station (cell tower) and other microwave sources used in mobile communications.

Polymerase

The enzyme Polymerase I, which has as one of its functions the repair of damage caused to DNA, as well as its replication, has its action interfered with by electromagnetic waves and mutations can occur.

Myasthenia

Myasthenia, a disorder of neuromuscular transmission that leads to fluctuating weakness and abnormal tiredness and fatigue, is attributed to the blockade of acetylcholine receptors as a consequence of radiation.

Polymyositis

Mild polymyositis may also occur. This relatively uncommon inflammatory disease entails weakness, swelling, sensitivity and damage to the muscles, belonging to the group of myositis.

How Folates Affect Epigenetics

There are three nutritional factors that affect epigenetics more than others in different ways: folates, methionine and S-adenosylmethionine

(SAMe). "These have a very powerful impact on it."

Folates are promoters of serotonin reuptake. However, even if a person is undermethylated and has an activity-related problem with low serotonin levels, such as depression or anxiety, folates should not be given. The reason for this is that if you provide them, your methylation will improve and the patient will actually get worse.

The reason it could get worse is because, in epigenetic terms, folates act as deacetylase inhibitors and have much lower serotonergic activity.

Most people with autism will not have a serotonin problem and will improve with methyl folate. However, 10% of autistic children and adults have a problem with serotonin levels, and will have a severe decline if given methyl folate.

According to one report: "We've seen thousands of patients who had undermethylation depression. I've seen over 3,000 cases of clinical depression. I have this huge database. The biggest phenotype... is undermethylation. But if I gave them any form of folate , they would get worse. Their methylation would improve, they would get worse, because it has a dramatic impact on serotonin reuptake. In contrast, methionine and SAMe are natural serotonin reuptake inhibitors. Basically, they do the same thing as Prozac and Paxil, but folates "They have the opposite effect.

The latter are wonderful if you want to reduce the level of dopamine in people who suffer from schizophrenia or people who have high levels of anxiety - overmethylated people - which seems contradictory because folates are excellent methylating agents."

To reiterate, some undermethylated people are intolerant to folates, and some overmethylated people thrive on folates even though folates improve methylation.

CHAPTER 10

EPIGENETICAL DAMAGES FROM FOOD ADDITIVES

Not all additives are harmful, although we would like them not to be necessary. In social ideology there is the belief that they are there to contaminate us and that large companies have no scruples when it comes to incorporating them into food. This is not the case, and the purpose is the opposite: they are incorporated so that we can put foods free of potentially dangerous organisms and substances into our mouths.

The biggest problem is that its negative effect takes many years to manifest, since millions of consumers are needed to be able to evaluate its safety. Among the worst accepted are colorings, preservatives and flavor enhancers. We always think that food should not be used and should be shown in its natural state, an ecological utopia, since the only natural food is only that which we grow and eat immediately after collecting it. From there, the deterioration begins.

A good suggestion is to eliminate as much as possible, at least, processed foods, packaged foods and especially those with a long shelf life. It is also important to cook and eat fresh, prepared foods whenever possible.

Perhaps in a candy full of sugar it is not precisely the sugar that is harmful, but rather the colorings that are added to give it an attractive color. For example, if peppermint candies didn't have green dye, they would be a dirty white, never green.

There are dyes, for example, that have a good reputation, for example the natural dyes of caramel (150a-d), beet red (162), chlorophyll (140,141) and beta carotene (160a).

Here are 6 food colorings that can cause negative reactions in the body:

Orange Yellow (E110), Quinoline Yellow (E104), Carmoisine (E122), Allura Red (E129), Tartrazine (E102), Ponceau 4R (E124).

We can find them in: Popsicles, chocolate, sweet drinks, liqueurs, sports drinks, liqueurs, donuts, muffins, cookies, cakes, flavored milks, medicines and ice creams.

Among the problematic preservatives:

1. Sorbates, which are used to inhibit the growth of molds and yeasts that can cause them to spoil. Potassium sorbate is unlikely to be dangerous. Others, such as Sorbic acid 200, Sodium sorbate 201, Potassium sorbate 202 and Calcium sorbate 203, are added to cottage cheese, yogurt, dried meat, dried fruits, pickles, sweet wines, apple cider, flavored syrups and toppings. They are also widely used in pharmaceutical products, such as syrups, eye and nose drops, contact lens solution, and many

herbal supplements. And also in soaps, shampoos, moisturizing creams, anti-aging creams, hand creams, eye shadow, mascara, blushes, hair dyes, cream-based concealers and other liquid products.

2. Benzoates occur naturally in cranberries and other berries, vegetables, peppers, herbs, spices, mint, and honey. Both natural and added, they can cause sensitivity to foods and drinks such as non-cola soft drinks, liqueurs, and orange and fruit juices.

3. Sulfites (sulfur-containing preservatives). They are used in wineries to destroy undesirable bacteria in the containers in which the wine is stored as well as to prevent its deterioration. They can cause problems in asthmatic patients one or two minutes after consumption. Among them sodium and potassium metabisulfite, and sulfur dioxide (220).

They are present in dried apricots, dried apples, fresh fruit salad, liqueurs, juices, fruit juices, dried vegetables, pickled vegetables (such as onions and gherkins), hot sauces, sausages, vinegar, beer and wine, especially draft white. .

4. Propionates occur naturally in many foods and are usually caused by certain bacteria, as occurs for example in Swiss cheeses.Commonly added to breads, pies, pastries as a mold inhibitor. Calcium Propionate 282 is the most common and is used in humid environments to prevent mold from forming on bread.

5. Nitrites. They can convert to nitrosamines in the body and cause cancer. They are added to cooked ham, bacon, corned beef, salamis, hot dogs, sausages, cured and canned sausages.

6. Citric Acid. Prevents the growth of bacteria and gives foods a characteristic citrus/sour flavor. It is sometimes produced naturally or chemically (E3309).

Commonly added to cakes, cookies, soups, all types of sauces, packaged frozen products, canned foods, candy, jams and ice cream.

7. Flavor enhancers that can only be harmful at high doses or combined with amines and salicylates. Glutamates (622, 623, 624 and 625) are usually used.

They are added to soups, sauces, broths, condiments, Asian and vegetarian dishes, flavored chips, snacks, instant noodles.

8. The following list refers to food additives that have a negative influence on health and/or behavior. Dyes: 102, E107, 110, 122-129, 132, 133, 142, 150, 151, 155, 160b, Preservatives: 200, 210-213, 220, 221-227, 228, 249-252, 280-283, Antioxidants: 310-312, 319-321, Emulsifiers: 407, 413, 416, 421, Anti-caking agents: 553, Flavor Enhancers: 621, 622, 627, E634, 635, Various additives: E905, 925, 926, 1201, 1520, Artificial Sweeteners : 950, 951, E951, 952, 954.

CHAPTER 11

DISEASES AND NUTRITION

Both the environment and individual lifestyle can interact directly with the genome to influence epigenetic change. The most influential changes seem to be chemical and electromagnetic pollution, as well as intense mental disturbances. Once again we would have to leave biology and genetics, and reach physics and environmental chemistry, without forgetting psychology, to be able to understand these changes and how they influence.

These changes can be reflected at various stages throughout a person's life and even in later generations. For example, prenatal and early postnatal environmental factors influence the adult risk of developing several chronic diseases and behavioral disorders.

Cancer was the first human disease linked to epigenetics. According to studies conducted in 1983, using primary human tumor tissues, they found that the genes of colorectal cancer cells were substantially hypomethylated compared to normal tissues. This DNA hypomethylation can activate oncogenes and initiate chromosomal instability, while DNA hypermethylation can stably alter gene expression in cells as they divide.

An accumulation of genetic and epigenetic errors can transform a normal cell into an invasive or metastatic tumor cell.

So epigenetic changes can be used as biomarkers for the molecular diagnosis of early cancer.

There is several evidence showing that loss of epigenetic control over complex immunological processes contributes to autoimmune disease, especially lupus and even rheumatoid arthritis, through the overexpression of methylation-sensitive genes.

Likewise, epigenetic errors also play a role in the development of psychiatric, autistic, and neurodegenerative disorders in adults. Schizophrenia, for example, and mood disorders alter the formation of gamma-aminobutyric acid (GABA), while hypermethylation represses the expression of Reelin (a protein necessary for normal neurotransmission, memory formation and synaptic plasticity) in the brain tissue of patients with schizophrenia, bipolar illness and psychosis. Also, aberrant methylation mediated folate levels has been suggested as a factor in Alzheimer's disease. Findings in autopsy of brain tissue from patients with autism have revealed that it could be a consequence of reduced expression of several relevant genes.

The increase in knowledge and technologies in epigenetics over the last ten years allows us to better understand the interplay between epigenetic change, gene regulation and human diseases, and will lead to the development of new approaches for molecular diagnosis and treatments. .

Epigenetic modifications and cardiovascular diseases

The role of epigenetic changes in cardiovascular diseases could explain the determinants of the heritability of complex diseases, such as atherosclerosis, hypertension, metabolic syndrome and diabetes, which to date have not been explained by genetic studies of variation of sequence. In a recent study, the influence of parental origin on the association of the disease was examined and it was shown that the origin of a parent alters the risk. Therefore, these findings suggest that other non-sequence-dependent variations may contribute to heritable traits. It is important to review the relationships between epigenetics and genetics, epigenetics and nutrition, and how these relationships may influence cardiovascular disease. Together, these findings support the concept that epigenetic modifications can influence risk in complex diseases.

Importantly, epigenetic programming plays a crucial role in regulating pluripotency genes, which become inactive during differentiation. Among the mechanisms, the role of long-term stable epigenetic modifications that involve DNA methylation stands out.

No less important are the role of nutritional and environmental challenges in generational inheritance and epigenetic modifications, focusing on examples that are related to complex cardiovascular diseases and specifically analyzing the mechanisms by which homocysteine modifies epigenetic marks. Finally, and most importantly, the possibilities of modifying therapeutically acquired epigenetic tags are studied, summarizing currently available agents and speculating on future directions.

Nutrition and environment

The hypothesis is that environmental factors in crucial periods of early life (during fetal development, for example) may influence the risks of cardiovascular and metabolic diseases later in life. This concept is supported by a series of studies that have associated low birth weight in human populations with increased risk of cardiovascular disease.

Exposure to maternal hypercholesterolemia during gestation has been associated with increased incidence and accelerated progression of lesions in humans, rabbits, and mice. Exposure to different behavioral patterns during early postnatal life has also been shown to influence epigenetic modifications in experimental animal models. Therefore, it has been suggested that these long-lasting changes arise, at least in part, from epigenetically mediated alterations in gene expression that occur very early in life.

Applying these concepts to human populations, it has recently been proposed that social and environmental stresses during development may influence epigenetic processes that contribute to health disparities in cardiovascular diseases such as hypertension, diabetes, stroke, and diseases. coronaries.

More recent studies in animal models have begun to characterize epigenetic modifications that are influenced by the intrauterine environment. For example, feeding a low-protein diet to pregnant rats causes low birth weight, hypertension, and endothelial dysfunction in the offspring.

Studies have demonstrated a role for the renin-angiotensin system in this phenotype as treatment of pregnant mothers with angiotensin-converting enzyme inhibitors or angiotensin receptor (AT1R) antagonists alleviates hypertension in the offspring. Consistent with these previous results, offspring of pregnant mothers fed low-protein diets were found to have hypomethylated genes, along with increased adrenal expression of AT1bR (a protein), suggesting a role for specific hypomethylation in the regulation of elevated blood pressure in this model.

Other studies have reported that a low protein diet during pregnancy in the rat results in overexpression of hepatic glucocorticoid receptors.

It has been shown that supplementation of a protein-restricted maternal diet in rats with methyl groups by adding folate or glycine decreases hypertension and improves endothelium-dependent vasodilation. These data support the hypothesis that folate may influence fetal development and the risk of cardiovascular disease in the next generation. Interestingly, providing folate to offspring, rather than pregnant mothers, increased the methylation status of some, but not all, of the genes modified by maternal protein restriction, suggesting that some epigenetic modifications may not be reversible by nutritional interventions in the offspring.

Nutrition in pregnancy

Several experts have insisted that environmental factors in crucial periods of early life (during fetal development, for example) can influence the risks of cardiovascular and metabolic diseases later in life. This concept is supported by a series of studies that have associated low birth weight in human populations with increased risk of cardiovascular disease. As we have noted, individuals exposed prenatally to famine during the Dutch winter of 1944 experienced a higher prevalence of obesity and coronary heart disease in adulthood than those born after that period. The studies found that low-weight newborns had a higher risk of coronary heart disease later in life and that increasing birth weight was associated with a gradual decrease in risk.

It has also been shown that exposure to different behavioral patterns during postnatal life influences epigenetic modifications. Therefore, it has been suggested that these long-lasting changes arise, at least in part, from epigenetic alterations in gene expression that occur early in life.

Likewise, if we apply these concepts to human populations, it is likely that social and environmental stresses during childhood development can influence epigenetic processes, more than genetics itself.

This would explain health disparities in relation to cardiovascular diseases such as hypertension, diabetes, and coronary heart disease.

More recent studies have begun to characterize epigenetic modifications that are influenced by the intrauterine environment.

For example, feeding a low-protein diet to pregnant women causes low birth weight, hypertension, and endothelial dysfunction in the offspring. Studies have demonstrated a role for the renin-angiotensin system in this phenotype, as treatment of pregnant mothers with angiotensin-converting enzyme inhibitors or angiotensin receptor antagonists alleviates hypertension in the offspring. Consistent with these previous results, the offspring of pregnant mothers fed low-protein diets were found to have hypomethylated genes and consequent elevated blood pressure.

Other studies have reported that a low-protein diet during pregnancy results in overexpression of the hepatic glucocorticoid receptor. These studies established an underlying epigenetic mechanism, which would give rise to a large number of metabolic pathways involved in the pathology of numerous diseases, including obesity, diabetes and atherosclerosis.

CHAPTER 12

EPIGENETIC ANALYSIS

According to an article published in Nature Biotechnology, it has been shown that epigenetic tests have the same technical quality and rigor as genetic tests, obtaining very similar results in all cases, and a reliability similar to genetic analyzes routinely used in studies. hospitals.

The international validation of epigenetic tests will allow progress in their clinical implementation, and they can be used to early detect tumor DNA circulating in the blood, evaluate samples archived in pathological anatomy laboratories for years, contribute to establishing credible epigenetic patterns that analyze differences between healthy tissue and with different diseases or, that the obtaining of complete epigenomes with each of the 6,000 million bricks that make up the human genome even begins to spread.

For a long time, it was assumed that paternal epigenetic marks are completely erased after the fusion of sperm and eggs, but we now know that some paternal DNA methylation probably survives this process. Even a temporary change in maternal diet can cause difficulties in learning skills in offspring, particularly affecting the ability to adequately learn a spatial navigation task.

Epigenetics is regulated by environmental factors and this can be transmitted from generation to generation, since the DNA of eggs and sperm is also regulated epigenetically. Epigenetics dilutes the classic border between genetic factors and environmental factors, and assumes they are interrelated. So much so, that epigenetic tests can be used to predict the risk of suffering from a certain disease or predict the response to a certain drug.

For all these reasons, the analysis of methylation patterns throughout the genome in sick patients and the comparison of these with those present in healthy individuals has become a potential tool for the diagnosis of diseases with clinically relevant phenotypes.

Why analyze it in hair?

Hair, as a reservoir tissue, provides many advantages to serum or urine analysis. It grows one cm each month, and for example, a 2 cm lock of hair will therefore reflect the level of trace elements of the last two months. Allows the sample to be sent by mail without special conditions. In contrast, serum mineral analysis reflects a specific situation, that of the moment of extraction, and the result does not reflect the nutritional status.

Urine analysis can be useful to measure the elimination profile of toxic elements in occupational hygiene or to measure the elimination rate of Ca, P and Mg in relation to bone metabolism, but not to evaluate nutritional status. Hair, in addition, is one of the best samples to preserve and transport good quality DNA, although for it to be correct, the hair must have the attached hair follicle or root, clean and thick. These hairs normally contain hair follicles, or bulbs, in which there is living tissue from which DNA can be extracted and the presence of a large number of elements can be observed. Hair samples are best preserved dry, in sealed, wax-free envelopes. Properly sealed and labeled envelopes can be stored in a dry container or in a plastic bag with silica gel or some other drying agent. Wax-free envelopes are porous, which allows the sample to remain ventilated.

Through this test, we will analyze:

Whether you are healthy or suffering from an illness, this analysis will show you the body's tendency and internal needs (impossible to detect by other means, such as a simple blood test).

There are accurate indicators of vitamins, minerals, essential fatty acids, amino acids. Also, indicators of toxins (heavy metals, chemicals...). Microbiology indicators (fungi, parasites, viruses, bacteria...) EMF and ELF indicators (computer radiation, electrical network, mobile radiation...)

Nutritional condition:

Evaluation of deficiency states due to malnutrition, weight loss diets, malnutrition, poor absorption and syndromes related to gastrointestinal disorders, age-related deficiency situations, pharmacological treatments and various pathologies.

Among others, we will find:

MACROMINERALS

Calcium, Phosphorus, Magnesium...

MICROMINERALALS and TRACE ELEMENTS

Iron, Copper, Zinc, Manganese, Selenium, Cobalt, Nickel, Vanadium, Silicon, Chromium, Selenium Molybdenum...

TYPICAL RELATIONSHIPS

Ca/Mg, Ca/Fe, Ca/Zn, Fe/Cu, Zn/Cu...

Toxic Elements:

It is used to evaluate long-term exposure to toxic elements that represent health risks, both due to their diffusion in the environment and in the work environment. These elements can progressively damage various neurological enzymatic processes, or affect different systems in our body. Among others:

Aluminum, Lead, Arsenic, Mercury, Cadmium, Barium...

CHAPTER 13

NATURAL TREATMENTS

Much of the search for anti-aging substances has focused on external appearance such as graying hair, wrinkles and sagging muscles. However, aging is much more than physical changes in our body's appearance. While "feeling old" may be a state of mind as well as a set of physical sensations, the aging process itself is a biological consequence.

The changes due to aging in our cells, muscles and hearing, as well as those in the immune system, appear to be irreversible, but they can be slowed down with human colostrum due to the growth factors it contains. These growth factors stimulate our skeletal system and muscle development at the cellular level, by regulating metabolism.

Although the theory about telomeres and longevity seems very new, natural medicine had already studied the secret of "eternal youth" hundreds of years ago without having to resort to complicated conclusions or sophisticated laboratory methods. Current medical science has only confirmed what we already knew, which is no small merit.

In my book Anti-aging medicine published in 2009, and later in Telomeres, anti-aging biology,

I already described in great detail all the physical and psychological processes that induce aging in us, as well as the solutions that alternative medicines provide to delay and even reverse it. I refer the interested reader to review them, if they wish to expand their thirst for knowledge.

In this chapter I will talk only about those natural substances that have a proven action on the stability and structure of telomeres, in addition to the general aging processes, an effect that is already being evaluated and confirmed by the most prestigious researchers. As they are natural, organic products, they can be consumed on a daily basis without apparent dangers to health, although it is better to have the help of an expert. Success will depend on its continuity, because when it comes to aging we must keep in mind that we always fight against the time factor and it does not stop.

Finally, when we modify our organic response to external elements using appropriate natural products, we are influencing the altered epigenetic data that caused damage to DNA and gene expression.

NATURAL SUBSTANCES

Just because you can manipulate genes for happiness doesn't mean you can ignore lifestyle factors, as that would be unwise. The basic fundamentals are still important - healthy eating, enjoyable exercise, restful sleep, rewarding work, etc.

Research suggests that the modern diet is increasingly low in several important nutrients that have a direct impact on aging and our brains are suffering thanks to this situation.

The following relationship is the most relevant and is now the subject of study and application by doctors and specialists in alternative medicines.

PLANTAS MEDICINALES

ASTRAGUS (Astragalus gallinaceus)

Other names: Huang Qi, Bei Qi, Hwanggi, Milk Vetch.

Astragalus is a plant native to Asia whose name means "yellow leader", since the root is yellow and is considered one of the most important herbs in traditional Chinese medicine, often combined with other herbs to strengthen the body. against diseases.

Parts used:

The dried root.

Composition:

Astragaloside IV and cycloastragenol. Simple sugars, polysaccharides, saponins, flavonoids, 21 amino acids (including asparagine, alanine, proline, arginine, aspartic acid), riboflavin, folic acid, vitamin P, organic acids, coumarin, sitosterol, daucosterol, choline and betaine. Also isoflavones, iron, manganese, zinc, rubidium and selenium.

Medical uses:

Recent research in China suggests that because astragalus is an antioxidant, it may help people with severe forms of heart disease, relieve symptoms and improve heart function.

It can also be a mild diuretic and behaves as an adaptogen, a substance that helps protect the body against various types of stress, including physical, mental, pathogenic or environmental.

It contains antioxidants, which protect cells against damage caused by free radicals, byproducts of cellular energy, helping to protect the body against diseases such as cancer and diabetes.

It is used to protect and support the immune system, for the prevention of colds and respiratory infections, to reduce blood pressure, and to protect the liver.

It has antibacterial and anti-inflammatory properties and also topically on the skin of wounds. Additionally, studies have shown that it has antiviral properties.

In the United States, researchers have looked at astragalus as a possible treatment for people whose immune systems are weakened by chemotherapy or radiation. In these studies, astragalus supplements appear to help people recover faster and live longer. Research on the use of astragalus for people with AIDS has had mixed results.

Action on telomeres:

Marketed, astragalus extract is advertised as a telomerase activator, as it converts into the hTERT gene that activates the telomerase enzyme. The molecule cycloastragenol present in the root seems to be the most important active part.

In summary:

Adaptogen: protects the body against stress and illness.

Anemia: A recent study suggests it may improve blood counts in people with aplastic anemia.

Colds and flu: In traditional Chinese medicine, astragalus is used as part of an herbal combination to prevent or treat colds. Animal tests suggest it may act against cold viruses.

Diabetes: Astragalus appears to lower blood sugar.

Fatigue or lack of appetite from chemotherapy: Some studies suggest that astragalus may help reduce the side effects of chemotherapy.

Heart diseases: Astragalus can act as an antioxidant and helps treat heart diseases.

Hepatitis: A combination of herbs containing astragalus to treat hepatitis has provided mixed results.

Kidney disease: It may help protect the kidneys and treat kidney disease, although the research is preliminary.

Seasonal allergies: May help reduce symptoms in people who have allergic rhinitis or hay fever.

Available shapes:

Astragalus can be available in a variety of forms:

Tincture (liquid alcohol extract)

Capsules and tablets, standardized and non-standardized.

Dried and powdered plant.

Topically for the skin.

Injectable forms are used in hospital or clinical settings in Asian countries.

Precautions:

At recommended doses, astragalus has no serious side effects and can generally be used safely.

High doses can interfere with the immune system.

Astragalus should not be given to a child with a fever because the herb can make the fever last longer or be stronger.

There is not much evidence about whether astragalus is safe for women who are breastfeeding.

Possible interactions:

With medications that suppress the immune system, such as cyclophosphamide.

Autoimmune diseases such as rheumatoid arthritis or lupus.

Lithium. Astragalus can make it more difficult for the body to get rid of the medicinal lithium, causing poisoning.

MILK THISTLE (Silybum marianum)

Parts used:

The seeds are used.

Composition:

Silymarin, silybin, histamine and flavonoids.

Medical uses:

It is the best known hepatoprotector, capable of regenerating the hepatocyte. It is also effective as a cholagogue, antitoxic, digestive and aperitif. It is used successfully in cirrhosis, bile insufficiencies, poor digestion and as a hypertensive tonic.

It has positive actions on digestive, nasal and vaginal bleeding.

Relieves flu, cystitis, migraines, allergies, and helps eliminate kidney and gallbladder stones.

Other uses:

Its synergy occurs with the dandelion. It is effective for motion sickness and vomiting during travel.

Good effects are attributed to it as a cardiotonic and in venous insufficiency.

It has an antioxidant effect 10 times greater than vitamin E, also helping to reduce cholesterol levels. Acts as an antihemorrhagic in liver failure.

Toxicity:

It has no toxicity.

Cellular anti-aging effect:

Silymarin present in milk thistle increases telomerase activity, while reducing it in cancer cells. This leads us to consider its role as an effective anti-aging agent by inhibiting endothelial progenitor cells.

The experiments examined whether silymarin, due to its hepatoprotective and antioxidant effect, can protect against senescence. To test this, mononuclear cells were isolated from the peripheral blood of healthy volunteers and cultured in a medium rich in rapamycin, with or without silymarin. It was soon seen that in the presence of silymarin, telomerase activity increased threefold, reducing the number of senescent cells and increasing proliferative activity. On the other hand, the reconstructive capacity was restored.

A synergy between iron and telomerase was also detected under the action of silymarin, significantly increasing lymphocyte proliferation.

One of the components of milk thistle, silibinin, actually decreases the activity of telomerase in cancer cells, inhibiting the activity of the enzyme and the secretion of prostate-specific antigen in prostate cancer cells.

Androgen-sensitive prostate cancer is very sensitive to dihydrotestosterone (DHT)-dependent telomerase activity, in turn decisive for cell immortality. However, telomerase activated by silymarin only seems to be inhibited in the case of malignant cells, and never in healthy ones, being stimulated in the latter case by silybinin.

So, in summary, silibinin can be used as an antiproliferative agent in prostate cancer, but additional benefits are achieved against some of the diseases associated with human aging.

And in relation to aging disorders, we know that milk thistle mitigates oxidative stress and improves memory.

GINKGO BILOBA

It is the only specimen of the Ginkgoaceae family. Specimens are recognized in the Tertiary and it is considered a unique living fossil. Originally from China and Japan, where it was a sacred tree that adorned palaces and temples, it is now spread throughout Europe.

It has a diameter of 2 meters and reaches 30 meters in height.

Parts used:

The leaves are used.

Composition:

Anthocyanins, flavonoids and ginkgolides.

Medical uses:

Excellent venotonic for varicose veins and hemorrhoids. It improves cerebral circulation, circulatory insufficiency and capillary fragility, being especially important in the elderly.

It behaves as a powerful antioxidant, increasing the amount of oxygen available to the brain, while preventing excessive blood clotting. It is believed that Ginkgo can also help improve the transmission of information in brain cells and reaction time in memory tests, being especially effective in Alzheimer's patients.

Other uses:

Effective in erectile dysfunction due to an increase in blood volume in the corpora cavernosa of the penis, also acting as a moderate antidepressant.

Gingko biloba extract can delay the onset of cellular senescence by activating P13k/Akt signaling pathways that increase telomerase activity.

Toxicity:

It has no toxicity, but may increase the action of anticoagulant medications. Do not ingest it 15 days before surgery.

MISTLETOE (Viscum album)

We find it attached to apple trees, poplars, oaks and other species. It is a protected species and is not always available for sale.

Parts used:

The leaves are used.

Composition:

Acetylcholine, inositol, mannitol, choline, viscalbin, saponin, vitamin C and mineral salts.

Medical uses:

Hypotensive, spasmolytic and antitumor. It is a very effective remedy for all tumor processes, especially those that settle in the head. Some specialists apply it in situ, through injections, which allows higher doses to be used and localized tumors to dissolve better. It is also used effectively in hypertension, arteriosclerosis and tinnitus.

Other uses:

It has antiepileptic and diuretic effects. It has synergy with the olive tree in hypertension. Its ability to protect against the effects of oxidative stress and antiaging potential have been shown to improve the production of nitric oxide (NO) and reduce the effects of free radicals.

It produces an increase in cell viability and prevents premature cell aging.

Toxicity:

Its degree of toxicity is medium. Take it with medical advice.

GREEN TEA (Camellia sinnensis)

The part of the plant used for therapeutic purposes is the leaves.

Composition:

Polyphenols and catechins. Also caffeine, vitamins B, C, E, K, P, U and F, chlorophyll, minerals, pectin, saccharides, amino acids, butyric acid and saponins. The amount of catechin tends to increase as the season progresses and thus, the first spring crop contains 12-13% catechin (13-17% as tannin), while the summer tea (third crop) contains 13 - 14% (17-21% as tannin). This explains why summer's second and third crop teas are more astringent.

Black, green, Oolong and white teas are prepared from the same leaves and the difference is in the harvesting, drying, fermentation and roasting. Green tea and black tea have the highest concentrations of active catechins, since they do not go through this process. Still, catechins represent 80 percent of the polyphenolic flavonoids present in green tea, while in black tea they represent approximately 20 percent to 30 percent.

The most important active ingredient in terms of its action on telomerase is catechins (EC, ECG, EGC and EGCg), from the flavonoid family. Epigallocatechin gallate (EGCG) is the most powerful of these catechins, with antioxidant activity approximately 25-100 times more potent than vitamins C and E.

A cup of green tea provides 10-40 mg of polyphenols and has antioxidant effects comparable to a serving of broccoli, spinach, carrots or strawberries.

Green tea polyphenols, including EGCG (epigallocatechin gallate) and many others, have been found to offer protection against several types of cancer. The polyphenols in green tea can make up up to 30 percent of the leaf's dry weight, so when you drink a cup of green tea, you're drinking a pretty potent solution of healthy polyphenols.

Green tea is the least processed type of tea, so it also contains the highest amounts of EGCG than all other tea varieties.

Keep in mind, however, that many green teas are oxidized, and this process can remove many of their valuable properties.

The best sign to look for when evaluating the quality of a tea is its color: if the green tea is brown instead of green, it is most likely oxidized.

It has favorable effects on telomeres.

Medical uses:

Traditional Chinese Medicine has always known about the medicinal benefits of green tea. Just as grapes and wine were spread throughout the world initially by the Phoenicians and later by other traders, tea was later introduced to Western countries by those same traders and travelers.

The health benefits provided by green tea are very similar to those described for resveratrol from the grape seeds that give rise to red wine.

It has antioxidant, anticancer, anti-inflammatory, thermogenic, probiotic and antimicrobial properties. It is used in muscular dystrophy, heart disease, and to slow the development of tumors in general by inhibiting the action of urokinase.

Research has shown that green tea can help improve the quality of the arterial wall by lowering lipids.

The most promising experiments are its ability to protect against experimentally induced DNA damage, and slow or stop the initiation and progression of unwanted cell colonies.

Other studies show evidence that it provides immunoprotective qualities, particularly for patients undergoing radiation or chemotherapy. The white blood cell count in these people shows that there is a big difference between those who consume green tea, compared to those who do not.

Being a tea made from fresh leaves, unfermented tea; The oxidation of catechins is minimal, and therefore they are capable of acting as antioxidants. Researchers believe that catechin is effective because it easily binds to proteins, blocking bacteria from adhering to cell walls and inducing their destruction. It also reacts with toxins created by harmful bacteria and metals such as lead, mercury, chromium and cadmium, preventing liver damage.

Toxicity:

Those of caffeine.

NUTRIENTS

Vitamin D3

Vitamin D, although its name suggests, is not actually a vitamin, but rather a neuroregulatory steroid hormone, which has a marked influence on approximately 10 percent of all the genes in the body.

In a study of more than 2,000 women, those with higher levels of vitamin D had fewer aging-related changes in their DNA, as well as fewer inflammatory responses. These data were also confirmed in men, meaning that people with higher levels of vitamin D may actually age more slowly than people with lower levels of vitamin D.

Leukocyte telomere length (LTL) is a predictor of aging-related diseases. As you age, LTL becomes shorter, but if you have chronic inflammation, telomere length decreases much more quickly because the body's inflammatory response increases white blood cell volume. Vitamin D concentrations also decrease with age, while C-reactive protein (a mediator of inflammation) increases. This double effect increases the general risk of developing autoimmune diseases such as multiple sclerosis and rheumatoid arthritis.

The good news is that vitamin D is a powerful inhibitor of the body's inflammatory response, and by reducing inflammation, the volume of white blood cells is decreased, creating a positive chain reaction that can protect us against a variety of diseases. In essence, it protects the body from deterioration due to aging.

Researchers have discovered that subsets of leukocytes have receptors for the active form of vitamin D3, allowing the vitamin to have a direct effect on these cells. This may also explain the specific connection between vitamin D and autoimmune diseases.

The most favorable way to optimize vitamin D levels would be through safe sun exposure. We should emphasize, however, how superior vitamin D synthesized by the sun is compared to oral vitamin D.

Its deficiency negatively affects the following diseases:

Cancer, hypertension, heart disease, autism, obesity, rheumatoid arthritis, diabetes 1 and 2, multiple sclerosis, Crohn's disease, flu, colds, tuberculosis, septicemia, premature aging, psoriasis, eczema, insomnia, depression, muscle pain, cavities, periodontal disease, macular degeneration, myopia, seizures, fertility, asthma, migraines, cystic fibrosis, Alzheimer's disease and schizophrenia.

Optimal levels are 50-70 ng/ml. If you prefer oral vitamin D3, consume 800 to 1,000 IU/day which could be increased to 2,000 IU per day in individuals with obesity, osteoporosis, limited sun exposure (e.g., housebound or workers), or poor absorption.

If you use tanning beds, be sure not to expose yourself to harmful magnetic fields, such as those that use magnetic ballasts to generate light, using those that use electronic ballasts.

Vitamin D, until now preferably used for calcium metabolism, may have an effect on the length of leukocyte telomeres, preventing the rate of shortening. As we know, leukocytes are an extraordinary source of DNA, as are sperm, saliva and the hair follicle.

The researchers point out that vitamin D is a potent inhibitor of the pro-inflammatory response and slows down the turnover of leukocytes (LTL), whose length predicts the development of diseases related to aging, and its shortening decreases with each cell division and with the increased inflammation.

In one study, serum vitamin D concentrations were measured in 2,160 women, aged 18-79 years (mean age: 49.4). They divided the group into three parts, based on vitamin D levels, and found that older age was significantly associated with shorter leukocyte telomere length (LTL).

High serum levels of vitamin D were related to greater length, and this result held even after adjustment for age and other variables that could be independently affected, such as time of year, menopause, use of hormones. replacement, physical activity and sun exposure.

The LTL difference between the highest and lowest levels of vitamin D was highly significant and the authors stated that this was equivalent to 5 years of aging. It was concluded that high levels of vitamin D, easily modifiable through nutritional supplements, were associated with greater LTL (leukocyte telomere) length. This highlights the potentially beneficial effects of vitamin D on aging and age-related diseases. The relationship between moderate regular exercise and minimizing telomere erosion was also analyzed in both mice and humans.

One of the most widespread causes of the marked deficiency of vitamin D in the Western population is the abuse of sunscreens, with factors that already speak of total protection, or absolute blocking of ultraviolet rays. The rebirth of childhood rickets and the very high levels of osteoporosis and osteopenia are due to these blockers whose action, unfortunately, is not considered.

Exposure to the sun when it is below 50 degrees above the horizon does not provide any benefit from UVB rays (low intensity and does not pass through the glass), but it keeps us exposed to UVA rays, which due to their longer wavelength They can more easily penetrate the ozone layer and other obstacles (such as clouds and pollution, glass) on their way from the Sun to Earth.

We remember certain concepts: UVB rays penetrate less than UVA, but are more reflective; 90% are blocked by ozone and oxygen in the atmosphere, although it is more harmful to the biosphere. On the skin, it has a greater effect since it starts the effect quickly and then acts slowly and longer, giving the skin a tanned tone. It is essential for the synthesis of vitamin D and is filtered through glasses, clothing and sunscreens. Prolonged exposure depresses the immune system and ends up affecting the stratum corneum of the eye.

UVA rays, with a wavelength between 320 and 400 nm, easily reach the Earth's surface. It penetrates less deeply into the skin, but can cause redness, spots, lack of elasticity, dryness, premature wrinkles and skin aging.

These rays maintain the same intensity throughout the year, even on cloudy days, during all hours of the day. Even if the skin is tanned, it continues to absorb these rays that degrade collagen and elastin and cause alterations in melanin (stains). These types of rays are capable of passing through windows, light clothing or even the car windshield. In greenhouses, they are the key to plant development. They turn out to be the most dangerous, since since they do not damage the skin immediately, many people do not take care of them.

Under optimal environmental exposures, the body can produce about 20,000 IU of vitamin D per day by exposing the entire body; about 5,000 IU with 50 percent of the body exposed, and if you only expose 10 percent it will produce 1,000 IU.

In summary we can say that vitamin D favors the transport of calcium and phosphorus at the intestinal level, stimulates mineralization in the bones, promoting the biosynthesis and maturation of collagen. It mobilizes calcium into the fluid compartment of the bone (which explains the need for adequate hydration), in a manner similar to PTH (parathyroid hormone), maintaining muscle integrity by transferring calcium and phosphorus.

It also inhibits the secretion of PTH and has certain antitumor activity through the lymphomedullary system.

Latest research

Studies have linked vitamin D deficiency to many health problems including autoimmune diseases, cardiovascular disease, cognitive impairment, and cancer. In this sense, previous studies have shown that high levels of vitamin D - specifically 25-hydroxyvitamin D - is associated with a reduced risk of cancer.

A systematic review of seven studies at the annual conference of the Society for Endocrinology in Brighton (2016), showed that a deficiency of vitamin D creates an increased risk of developing cancer.

How to synthesize it

This essential fat-soluble nutrient is activated simply by exposing the body to the sun for a minimum of 5 to 30 minutes a day. However, it is not enough to expose yourself to the sun, since for the conversion of ergosterol into cholecalciferol (active form of vitamin D), sufficient fat reserves and eating equally fatty foods are needed. Currently, and due to the obsession against fat and weight loss diets, nine out of 10 Westerners do not meet their daily needs and do not eat enough foods that contain Vitamin D or precursors, such as egg yolks, fortified drinks or blue fish liver. The deficiency is more pronounced for people living in the northern parts of the planet, especially during the winter.

A dose of 1,000 IU of vitamin D3 is equivalent to one can of tuna, or 25 egg yolks, or eight cups of fortified beverage, or 25 cups of fortified cereal. In countries that have little sunlight, it would not be feasible to get enough Vitamin D through food alone. In the UK, one in five adults are deficient in vitamin D and three in five have low levels. During the winter, 75 percent of dark-skinned people are deficient. We must also remember that in hot countries, with a strong incidence of the sun, there are thousands of cases of rickets, which indicates that the sun is not the only factor in the metabolism of vitamin D.

In a recent study at the University Hospital and University of Warwick, with a total of 1,125 participants, 5 out of 7 showed low levels of vitamin D linked to an increased risk of cancer. In another separate experiment, researchers discovered that these people respond better to Vitamin D, improving their immune system.

BIOTIN (Vitamin H, vitamin B8)

Promotes a healthy nervous system, skin and muscles. The coenzyme acts in the metabolism of glucose and fats, helping in the utilization of proteins, folic acid, pantothenic acid, and Vitamin B-12. Promotes healthy hair.

Organic functions:

It has an important role as a coenzyme in the metabolism of carbohydrates, proteins and fats, intervening in numerous vital reactions, many of them only verifiable in animals. Among these actions are the catabolism of the amino acids leucine and isoleucine, the metabolization of Coenzyme A, the carboxylation of pyruvic acid, the formation of citrulline, an intermediate substance in the synthesis of urea, and the formation of aspartic acid, being a essential constituent in the formation of protoplasm.

It is also essential for the normal use of fats and certain albumins, and properties are attributed to it that strengthen the bronchi and lungs, intervening with nicotinic acid in the healing of Pellagra.

Some dependence on the supply of Biotin has been noted, especially in children.

In men, deficiency states can be found that have symptoms consisting of muscle pain and fatigue, together with seborrhea and furunculosis, which can degenerate into psoriasis.

Dermatitis is another characteristic feature of vitamin deficiency, which manifests as scaly, itchy, scaly, and greasy skin. There is depigmentation in the hair and skin, loss of skin around the eyes first and then throughout the body, with alterations being noticed in the genitals and embryonic malformations.

All of these alterations are very normal in animals but less common in humans, who usually suffer from benign dermatitis that quickly subsides with treatment. These pathologies focus on the extremities, they have a scaly, dry and grayish appearance and fatigue, apathy and anemia are normal.

In children there is seborrheic dermatitis, desquamative erythroderma and anemia, with certain physical and mental retardation appearing, with alopecia, conjunctivitis and defects in lymphocyte immunity.

Its deficiency produces alterations in the functioning of all the cells and tissues of the body, which manifest themselves in a marked decrease in energy in the brain that produces mood disorders, chronic fatigue and depression.

There is deterioration and hair loss, seborrheic, exfoliative dermatitis and eczema on the skin, and inflammation of the tongue (glossitis).

Biotin insufficiency also usually produces neuromuscular disorders such as myalgia and fibromyalgia, anemia, increased cholesterol, heart rhythm disturbances, depression of immune functions, alterations in digestion and metabolism, and congenital malformations.

Orthomolecular applications:

Premature aging.

Skin and hair alterations.

Prevents or relieves depression and apathy.

It intervenes in the formation of glucose from carbohydrates and fats, and helps insulin regulate blood sugar levels.

Influence on telomerase:

It increases endogenous RNA production, favoring genetic expression, which is why it probably reduces or reverses the rate of aging and the appearance of degenerative diseases.

It has an important role in the prevention of congenital malformations and probably in many genetic diseases.

ESSENTIAL FATTY ACIDS

Alpha-linolenic acid (AAL)

AAL has three main biological effects, which together contribute to its beneficial health effects.

1. It is a precursor to EPA and DHA in its effect to prevent the formation of blood clots. Its presence in colostrum and breast milk suggests that ALA plays a role in the growth and development of children. Likewise, it is important in preserving the health of the skin and hair of mammals.

2. Diets rich in ALA increase the content of total omega 3 fatty acids and phospholipids in the cell membrane. As the omega 3 content increases, the flexibility of the membranes and their ability to absorb and release nutrients increases.

3. ALA decreases inflammatory reactions by blocking the formation of compounds that

promote inflammation leading to arteriosclerosis and other chronic diseases.

Eicosapentaenoic acid (EPA)

EPA is the precursor of certain eicosanoids that tend to prevent inflammatory processes. EPA, not DHA, is responsible for the healthy effect of fish oil on triglycerides.

Docosahexaenoic acid (DHA)

DHA is an omega-3 fat that plays a very important role in keeping cell membranes healthy, flexible and resistant to oxidative stress, which decreases inflammation. Chronic inflammation is a key factor in many degenerative diseases, including dementia. Low levels of DHA have been linked to depression, memory loss, and even increased hostility, reflecting the importance of optimal brain function.

The Western diet is composed of many omega-6 fats and few omega-3 fats due to the heavy dependence on processed foods. DHA levels can be increased by eating more fish such as salmon and sardines, but currently most fish are contaminated with mercury and other toxic compounds, which is why many people prefer dietary supplements in pill form.

In fetuses and children, DHA is necessary for the development and maturity of the eyes, where they constitute 50% of the fatty acids in the retina, while they represent about 25% of the total fatty acids in the gray matter. of the brain.

Effects on telomeres:

A new study partially attributes longevity to consuming omega 3, which helps preserve DNA segments found in telomeres. Scientists essentially identify Omega 3 as a natural anti-aging nutrient.

Researchers at Ohio State University conducted tests on two different groups of people, one of them using omega-3 fatty acid supplements. Those who received the supplements had longer telomeres than those in the control group that received a placebo. There was also a 15 percent reduction in oxidative stress, somewhat higher than those who drank red wine and dark chocolate, two renowned antioxidants.

The conclusion is that the consumption of omega 3 fatty acids is a good additional system to help preserve telomere length, with the potential to reduce the risk of age-related diseases.

SELENIUM

The first experiments were done with animals and it was seen, as the most conclusive data, that it significantly prolonged life, more than anything due to its antioxidant action and its property to prevent coronary diseases. The only essential requirement for selenium to have these properties was that it be administered naturally (not from copper or sulfuric acid), from the earth (astragalus or walnuts) and that it be used for many years.

Its lack, on the contrary, caused premature aging, with differences being found between experimental animals of up to 25% greater longevity in those who took supplements.

But research on its functions was still unclear until an important fact was discovered: vitamin E, in order to perform its functions as an antioxidant, needed the presence of selenium; The synergy was a proven fact. The joint action of both nutrients managed to stop the harmful action of free radicals, which were capable of producing deadly chain reactions. Together with the fatty constituents of the cells, they multiply and obtain extra strength, which is stopped by antioxidants, among which is vitamin E.

Organic functions:

The way in which both substances act synergistically is believed to be concentrated in a specific enzyme called glutathione peroxidase, which accelerates the body's reactions, as long as it is protected by vitamin E.

Selenium is an antioxidant that protects vitamin E from degradation. It helps build the immune system by destroying free radicals, and in the production of antibodies. Selenium is stored in the liver, kidneys and muscles, and relatively low concentrations behave as a cancer preventive.

It also fortifies the energy cells of the heart, ensuring sufficient oxygen, helps eliminate arsenic, lead, mercury and cadmium, and when bound to glutathione peroxidase, protects tissues from the effects of oxidation.

The most demonstrated functions are these:

It is a powerful and effective antioxidant.

Maintains liver, heart and reproductive functions in good condition.

It collaborates in skin and tendon elasticity, as well as in the good condition of the joints.

It is necessary in the synthesis of prostaglandins, the formation of semen, the formation of coenzyme Q and nonspecific organic defenses.

Due to its antioxidant action, it prevents cancer, premature aging, skin and hair disorders, diabetes, as well as lack of muscle vigor.

Selenium is much more effective in conjunction with vitamins A, E and C, all powerful antioxidants. There are, however, some toxic forms of selenium on the market, such as sodium selenite, which is not recommended to be taken continuously and it is better to use the selenium-methionine mixture or brewer's yeast cultured in selenium.

Daily needs range between 0.05 to 0.15 mg, although 200 mcg are used in shock therapies.

Orthomolecular applications:

This therapy does not seek to cover the daily needs of selenium, but rather to apply it in higher doses for short periods, in order to achieve a rapid response in the body. The following are some valid experiences:

Premature aging, in conjunction with vitamins A, C and E.

Joint diseases, linked to copper.

Cardiovascular diseases, associated with vitamin E.

Progressive or traumatic muscular dystrophies, associated with vitamin E.

Atherosclerosis, high blood pressure or risk of atheromas.

Hair loss, along with vitamin B, zinc and silicon.

Liver cirrhosis.

As a preventative of cancer or in an early phase.

Frequent or serious infections, together with vitamins A and C.

Immunodeficiency syndrome.

Prostatitis and prostate adenoma, linked to zinc.

Hypothyroidism, along with the amino acid L-tyrosine.

Dermatitis or skin tumors.

Diseases that cause inflammatory processes.

Male infertility in association with zinc.

Heavy metal poisoning.

Little elasticity of muscles and tendons.

As a preventative of sudden infant death.

Incipient cataracts.

Cystic fibrosis.

Times of strong sports training.

As a corrector of the side effects of X-rays and ultraviolet radiation.

Medication, alcohol or drug poisoning.

To prevent poisoning from metal dental prostheses.

Toxicity:

Selenium itself is a very toxic mineral, but if we lack it the damage is also serious. It is best to take it in natural foods (garlic, wheat germ...) that are rich in it and if this is not possible, we can resort to dietary preparations.

The daily dose should be 25 mcg in infants, 100 mcg in children and 150 mcg in adults.

Overdose can be detected by the strong smell of garlic in the breath and sweat, hair loss, brittle nails, liver disease and skin rashes. Special care must be taken with industrial products that contain selenium, such as photocopiers, photoelectric cells, some paints and certain types of cement. Selenium-based shampoos and lotions that are recommended against dandruff are also common, and can be toxic if used continuously, since the skin absorbs the metal quite well.

A reddish pigmentation of the skin, anorexia, bad taste in the mouth, loss of sensitivity in the hands and fragile gums may be other symptoms of excess selenium.

OTHER IMPORTANT NUTRIENTS

Naturally, many other nutrients, although not all, have been studied in the dynamics of longevity, since only recently have researchers assumed that human beings could reach at least 120 years of life. However, I think it is possible to make some general recommendations based on the fact that most people are deficient in many of these key nutrients that we know are important for optimal health. Some, like astaxanthin and curcumin, have strong scientific support for their benefits.

Let's look at some of them that could help radically increase lifespan by protecting telomeres and possibly changing gene expression.

Astaxanthin (derived from Pluvialis Haematoccous microalgae)

In a 2009 study on multivitamin use and telomere length, telomere lengthening was also associated with the use of antioxidant formulas.

According to the authors, telomeres are particularly vulnerable to oxidative stress. Furthermore, inflammation induces oxidative stress and decreases telomerase activity.

Astaxanthin has emerged as one of the most potent beneficial antioxidants currently known, with potent anti-inflammatory capabilities and potential to protect DNA. Research has shown that it can protect against DNA damage induced by gamma radiation.

Among its unique features are:

It is without a doubt the most powerful antioxidant carotenoid when it comes to free radical scavenging, being 65 times more powerful than vitamin C, 54 times more powerful than beta-carotene and 14 times more powerful than vitamin E.

It is also much more effective than other carotenoids at "singlet oxygen blocking," which is a particular type of oxidation. In this aspect, it is 550 times more powerful than vitamin E, and 11 times more powerful than beta-carotene.

Astaxanthin crosses both the blood-brain barrier and the blood-retinal barrier (something beta-carotene and lycopene do not), providing antioxidant and anti-inflammatory protection for the eyes, brain, and central nervous system.

Another characteristic that makes astaxanthin different from other carotenoids is that it cannot function as a pro-oxidant.

Many antioxidants act as pro-oxidants (meaning they cause more oxidation rather than fighting it) when they are present in tissues in sufficient concentrations.

For this reason, it is not advisable to take many antioxidant supplements such as beta-carotene, for example. Astaxanthin, on the other hand, does not function as a pro-oxidant, even in high amounts, making it highly beneficial.

Finally, one of its most profound characteristics is its unique ability to protect the entire cell from damage, both the water-soluble part and the fat-soluble portion of the cell. Other antioxidants affect only one or the other portion. This is due to the unique physical characteristics of astaxanthin, which allow it to reside within the cell membrane, thus protecting the interior of the cell.

Ubiquinol (CoQ10)

Coenzyme Q10 (CoQ10) is the fifth most popular supplement in the United States, taken by 53 percent of Americans, according to a 2010 survey by ConsumerLab.com.

CoQ10 is used by every cell in your body through a substance known as ubiquinone or ubiquinol, which helps produce cellular energy and reduce the typical signs of aging. People over 25 years of age cannot convert oxidized CoQ10 to ubiquinol.

CoQ10 deficiency also accelerates DNA damage, and because coenzyme Q10 is beneficial for heart health and muscle function, depletion of it leads to fatigue, muscle weakness, pain and, eventually, heart failure. .

Although CoQ10 appears to improve quality of life, it does not significantly increase longevity.

Krill Oil

People who have an omega-3 fatty acid index of less than four percent age faster than people with indexes above eight percent. Therefore, the omega-3 index may also be an effective marker on the rate of aging.

According to Dr. Harris' research, omega-3 fats appear to play a role in activating telomerase.

The favorite omega-3 fatty acids from animal sources come from krill oil, as it has a number of benefits not found in other omega-3 fatty acid supplements such as fish oil.

In addition to having a high potential for contamination, fish oil supplements also have a higher risk of oxidation damage and rancidity.

Krill oil also contains naturally occurring astaxanthin, which makes it almost 200 times more resistant to oxidative damage compared to fish oil.

Vitamin K2

Vitamin K could be as important as vitamin D, as research continues to provide a growing number of health benefits. Although most people get enough vitamin K from their diet to maintain proper blood clotting, it is not enough to offer protection against more serious health problems.

For example, research has suggested over the past few years that vitamin K2 may provide substantial protection against prostate cancer, which is a leading cause of cancer among men in the United States.

The results of other research showed that the benefits of Vitamin K help boost heart health. In 2004, the Rotterdam Study, which was the first study to demonstrate the beneficial effect of vitamin K2, showed that people who consume 45 mcg of vitamin K2 daily live seven years longer than people who only ingest 12 mcg per day. day.

In a later study called Prospect Stud, 16,000 people were observed for 10 years. Researchers found that every additional 10 mcg of vitamin K2 in your diet resulted in a 9 percent decrease in cardiac events.

Vitamin K2 is present in fermented foods, especially cheese and the Japanese food natto, which is in fact the richest source of K2.

Magnesium

Magnesium also plays a very important role in the body's detoxification processes and is therefore important in helping to prevent damage caused by environmental chemicals, heavy metals and other toxins. Even glutathione, considered by many to be your body's most powerful antioxidant, along with SOD, requires magnesium for its synthesis.

Magnesium acts as a buffer between neuronal synapses, particularly those involved with cognitive functions (learning and memory). Magnesium integrates into the receptor without activating it and protects it from excessive activation by other neurochemicals, especially glutamate. Glutamate is the "excitoxin," which can damage the brain if it builds up, and magnesium helps prevent this buildup. This is why magnesium is often touted as a "soothing" nutrient.

Good sources of magnesium are whole organic foods, especially dark leafy green vegetables, seaweed, dried pumpkin seeds, unsweetened cocoa, flax seeds, butter, and whey.

A suitable magnesium supplement is magnesium threonate, particularly good due to its ability to penetrate cell membranes and cross the blood-brain barrier, which is important for preserving good cognitive functioning as you age.

According to the research presented, magnesium also plays an important role in DNA replication, repair and RNA synthesis, and dietary magnesium has been shown to have a positive correlation with increased telomere length.

Other research has shown that long-term deficiency leads to telomere shortening in rats and in cell cultures. Apparently, the lack of magnesium ions has a negative effect on the integrity of the genome. Insufficient amounts of magnesium also reduce your body's ability to repair damaged DNA, and can induce chromosomal alterations.

According to the authors, the hypothesis is that "magnesium influences telomere length is reasonable, as it affects DNA integrity and repair, in addition to its possible role in oxidative stress and inflammation."

Folate (Vitamin B9 or Folic Acid)

Folate helps prevent depression, compulsive disorders, brain atrophy, and other neurological problems. Folate deficiency is correlated with memory problems, slowed mental processes, and overall cognitive decline, particularly in older people. The body also needs folate to produce red blood cells and for them to reach the optimal size (MCV). Folate deficiency is thought to cause elevated levels of homocysteine, which may be one of the main factors in heart disease and Alzheimer's. However, recent studies could refute that idea.

It is useful for the prevention of depression, seizure disorders and brain atrophy. One of the unfortunate and avoidable reasons why some believe folate numbers are declining is due to the increasing prevalence of obesity, which negatively affects the way most people metabolize this important vitamin.

Many times, people confuse folate with folic acid and it is important to know the difference. Folate is a natural form of the vitamin and contains all the isomers the body needs for optimal functioning. Folic acid is the synthetic form of the vitamin that is used in most supplements and fortified foods.

Foods rich in folate include egg yolks, sunflower seeds, asparagus, avocados, broccoli, cauliflower, basil, parsley and green vegetables such as romaine lettuce, turnip greens, cabbage and spinach.

According to a study published in the Journal of Nutritional Biochemistry, plasma concentrations of folate (a B vitamin) correspond to the length of the telomere, both in men and women, so it has an important role in maintaining the integrity and DNA methylation, which influences the length of your telomeres.

B12 vitamin

Vitamin B12 is appropriately known as "the energy vitamin," and the body requires it for a number of vital functions. Among them: energy production, formation of red blood cells, DNA synthesis, and the formation of myelin, the insulation that protects nerve endings and allows them to communicate with each other.

Unfortunately, research suggests that a minimum of 25 percent of American adults are deficient in this vitally important nutrient, and nearly half of the population has suboptimal blood levels.

Vitamin B12 is found exclusively in animal tissues, including foods such as meat, beef liver, lamb, venison, salmon, shrimp, poultry and eggs. It is believed, therefore, that those who do not eat meat or animal products are at risk of deficiency, which is not true. This essential water-soluble vitamin is synthesized by the intestinal flora, with the help of gastric intrinsic factor and the trace element cobalt. Subsequently, it accumulates in the liver for a long time.

Vitamin A

According to the study published in the Journal of Nutritional Biochemistry, telomere lengthening is positively associated with dietary intake of vitamin A.

It plays an important role in the immune response, and if there are deficiencies, a predisposition to infections develops that can promote telomere shortening. However, you don't need large quantities. 50,000 IU a day is enough.

FOOD

CABBAGE (Brassica Oleracea) Cabbage

It is a plant that only produces leaves the first year and flowers appear in the second. It grows in humid, slightly fertile lands, rich in sulfur and calcium. You have to plant them spaced apart and this way they will resist the cold well. The soil must be prepared by plowing fifteen days before and the chosen fertilizers are already incorporated. If the climate is humid, it does not need watering.

It is harvested in autumn and winter and stored in a cold, dry place.

Composition:

It contains indole-3-carbinol, vitamins A, B, C and U, as well as iron and sulfur. Also calcium, magnesium, phosphorus, potassium, zinc and iodine.

Properties:

It is the best remedy against gastroduodenal ulcer, especially if we take it in the form of juice. It also helps to cure rheumatic diseases and liver diseases. However, it is difficult to digest and therefore its nutritional properties may be lost when cooking, so it is recommended not to throw away the broth. It is also suitable for chronic diseases of the respiratory tract, hoarseness and to disinfect the intestinal system, even from parasites.

The leaves can be used directly as a poultice to relieve rheumatic pain, low back pain, sciatica and neuralgia.

These poultices can also be used in bronchitis, liver congestion, cystitis, dysmenorrhea and prostatitis, as well as to ripen boils and cure varicose ulcers.

In the past, the juice was used to relieve ulcerated eyes, avoid discomfort due to excess food, and to correct the effect of alcohol.

Due to its lactic acid content, it disinfects the colon, although in this case it is better to use fermented cabbage. It also improves headaches, prevents cancer and can be applied externally to psoriasis, ulcers, bumps, boils, wounds and eczema.

The raw juice is taken for asthma, cystitis, bronchitis, neuralgia, against coughs and in gargles for throat irritations.

BROCCOLO (Brassica oleracea italica)

It is planted in the temperate season and the transplant is carried out when it reaches 15 cm in height, then leaving a distance of 60 cm between each plant. It needs a lot of water and it is necessary to protect it from frost and wind. It is harvested in the cold season, starting from the central part and then from the sides, otherwise the plant will be exhausted. The cuts will produce new shoots.

Composition:

It is rich in sulforaphane, vitamin A, calcium, phosphorus, iron, folic acid, potassium, magnesium, zinc, selenium and vitamins C and E, as well as indoles.

Properties:

It is used in medicinal applications similar to cabbage and cauliflower. It has interesting properties as an antioxidant, and its indole content gives it important anticancer properties, especially in estrogen-induced tumors.

The presence of sulforaphane makes it related to the fight against aging, by inducing proteasome activity and reducing the cellular accumulation of modified proteins. The proteasome enzyme allows the elimination of abnormal and unwanted cellular proteins, so its lack of activity induces cellular aging.

HOT CHILI (Chili Pepper)

Chili peppers contain capsaicin, the active ingredient in chili peppers and cayenne that give vegetables heat.

Therapeutic properties:

Reduces cholesterol levels by promoting its metabolism, increasing its degradation and excretion. In addition to reducing total blood cholesterol levels, reduced levels of capsaicinoids reduce LDL cholesterol, but do not affect HDL cholesterol levels.

Capsaicin blocks the action of a gene that causes arteries to constrict, allowing more blood to flow through the blood vessels.

With its consumption, a loss of body weight and an increase in the availability of some proteins responsible for metabolizing fats is observed.

In the long term, dietary consumption of capsaicin reduces blood pressure in hypertensive patients. It causes an increase in the production of nitric oxide, a gas molecule known to protect blood vessels against inflammation and dysfunction, as well as improving blood flow in the cavernous vessels of the penis.

It inhibits malignant cell proliferation, by reducing the activity of NADH oxidase – not the healthy reduced form – and suppresses its metabolic activation.

Induces apoptosis of tumor cells.

It has a hypoglycemic effect.

TURMERIC (Curcuma longa)

Perennial plant from the Cingiberaceae family that usually reaches one meter in height. It has 5 or 10 long-petiole leaves, white or yellow flowers and a large rhizome.

Composition:

Bitter principle, curcumin, resin, starch and organic acids.

Parts used:

roots and leaves

Medical uses:

It is used as a stomach tonic, as it stimulates the production of gastric juices, being suitable for whetting the appetite and for hypochlorhydria.

It is cholagogue, carminative and reduces cholesterol. It is a powerful anti-inflammatory.

Other uses:

It is part of the curry sauce, mixed with coriander, ginger, cumin, nutmeg and cloves.

Toxicity:

It has an anticoagulant effect.

Effects on cellular changes:

The research literature in relation to turmeric and cancer is truly enormous, demonstrating that there is clinical evidence on its properties to prevent and treat this disease. One of the investigations concluded with this report: "Curcumin (diferuloylmethane), a derivative of turmeric, is one of the most researched phytochemical substances, with multiple mechanisms showing that it can be an alternative to chemotherapy and to block side effects .

The pleiotropic role (effects of genes on traits) of this dietary compound includes the inhibition of cellular signaling pathways at various levels, such as transcription factors, enzymes, cell cycle arrest, proliferation, and alternative survival pathways. Curcumin prevents the production of cancer cells, as long as it is administered in sufficient doses. Currently, there is sufficient data to show that it intervenes favorably in phase II and phase III states in conditions such as multiple myeloma, pancreatic and colon cancer.

Curcumin acts as a powerful immune booster and anti-inflammatory. But perhaps its greatest value lies in its anti-cancer potential, and it is the one with the best evidence - based on literature and supported by its anti-cancer claims. Once it reaches cells, it affects more than 100 different pathways, including a key biological pathway necessary for the development of melanoma and other cancers.

The spice prevents laboratory strains of melanoma from proliferating and causes cancer cells to retreat, thereby shutting down factor kappa B (NF-kB), a powerful protein known to induce an abnormal inflammatory response that leads to a variety of disorders such as arthritis and cancer.

Curcumin can be used preventively or curatively, without its prolonged use generating new diseases or side effects. It has been shown to modulate the growth of tumor cells, preventing their ability to survive, without affecting healthy cells.

About telomeres

Various research has shown that curcumin increases the expression of telomerase and therefore helps preserve telomere length. To test this hypothesis, they looked at its effects on telomerase expression in brain cells exposed to beta-amyloid, a key source of oxidative damage and brain cell death linked to Alzheimer's disease. The researchers measured the effects of curcumin on cell survival and cell growth, intracellular oxidative stress, and telomerase expression in these brain cells. The results indicate that the protective effects of curcumin in Alzheimer's disease may be mainly due to its effects on telomerase expression. When the expression of telomerase was inhibited, the protective effects produced by curcumin disappeared.

GINGER (Zingiber officinale)

Recent research on epigenetics has revealed several of the already discussed aspects of ginger, especially its ability to impact chromatin and regulate epigenetic mechanisms, especially histone acetylation, a process by which an acetyl group undergoes for the molecule transfer.

Since we know that age, environment, lifestyle, and overall health can influence epigenetics, studies on this well-known culinary spice have now had scientific value.

The bottom line is that it is considered a potent herb with the ability to impact chromatin in the nucleus of a cell and regulate epigenetic mechanisms, particularly histone acetylation.

Acetylation is the process by which an acetyl group is transferred from one molecule to another, something that ginger - along with similar herbs such as turmeric, tulsi (holy basil) and cinnamon - have been shown to have an influence on regulating genetics.

One study supported the ability of ginger to increase histone H3 acetylation and suppress the expression of histone deacetylase 1 (HDAC1), removing the positive charge of histones and ultimately relaxing the structure of tightly bound chromatin, which It causes an increase in transcription - the first step in gene expression -, where a certain DNA strand is copied into RNA.

The enzymes that eliminate the acetyl trace are known as HDACs.

When a person consumes healthy foods like ginger, these epigenetic tags attached to histone proteins that surround DNA can be adjusted, which will influence the expression of genes that are linked to inflammatory and neuroprotective pathways.

Fresh or cooked ginger is the only way gingerol or shogaol will be found. Both are rapidly absorbed and serve to increase gastric tone and motility, as well as help relax intestinal muscles so that accumulated gas can be released.

SUPPLEMENTS

MELATONIN (N-acetyl-5-methoxytryptamine)

Recently, there has been an increase in research on melatonin, supporting Dr. Rosenzweig's theory that melatonin plays a critical role in aging. The results of these studies have uncovered several potential mechanisms of action to explain how melatonin affects aging and related diseases.

This substance, found in plants such as Chamomile and St. John's Wort, is secreted by the pineal gland thanks to the help of the amino acid tryptophan and serotonin, and is widely used to regulate sleep cycles and quality.

The first evidence implicating melatonin in aging is that its production by the pineal gland declines drastically with advancing age, which may explain the sleep disorders suffered by elderly people. Data indicate that peak nocturnal melatonin levels in humans are twice as high among young people (21-25 years old) as in middle-aged people (51-55 years old), and about four times higher in young people. than in older people (82-86 years).

Secretion during 24 hours is approximately twice as high at 20 years of age as at 60, in both men and women.

QUERCETIN

Quercetin is a flavonoid found in apples, onions, tea, red wine, and many other foods, as well as Ginkgo Biloba and St. John's Wort.

New reports explain that proteasome inhibition accelerates the onset of senescence in fibroblasts (cells that heal tissues and regenerate skin), and that this effect can be minimized by quercetin. The proteasome is an important cellular structure that degrades old or defective (e.g., oxidized) proteins. When its activity is decreased, an increase in aged cells is observed. The accumulation of oxidized elements and damage to cellular proteins cause the loss of proteasome activity.

Quercetin, and its fatty derivative quercetin caprylate, are potent proteasome activators. Furthermore, these compounds have a rejuvenating effect on middle-aged and senescent primary fibroblasts. When quercetin is added, fibroblasts maintain their useful life and maintain young morphology, its effect being more noticeable in old age, and less in very young people. The cells treated with both elements maintained their chromosomes with longer ends, as well as their original shape.

It was also surprising that in middle-aged and senescent people, the rate of cell proliferation was very high when quercetin or quercetin caprylate was applied for several weeks, although the effect began to be perceived in just 5 days.

Furthermore, the cells show a "rejuvenated phenotype" with more elongated morphology and a lower number of beta-galactosidase (a marker of senescence). Both quercetin and quercetin caprylate increase resistance to the cellular oxidative effect.

RESVERATROL

Resveratrol has achieved notorious fame as an antioxidant and anti-aging, just when wine had lost the market to beer. This fact should make us reflect on the role of resveratrol, an antioxidant present in red grapes and, consequently, in red wine. So we must be cautious in its assessment and take into account the scientific experiments carried out over a decade ago.

So and although my personal interest in resveratrol is pejorative, since I believe that it is a manipulation by wine sellers so that the population believes that it is a healthy drink, in an impartial position one can say the properties that they attribute to it, for example: it penetrates the center of the cell's nucleus, providing the right time for its DNA to repair the damage caused by free radicals. Research dating back to 2003 showed that resveratrol had the ability to increase the lifespan of yeast cells.

The results showed that resveratrol could activate a gene called sirtuin1, which is also activated during caloric restriction in several species. Since then, studies in nematode worms, fruit flies, fish, mice and human cells have linked resveratrol to the extension of their lifespan.

If you want to take resveratrol and don't want to consume wine, look for muscat grapes and eat them whole, with skin and seeds.

Resveratrol is a stilbenoid, a type of natural phenol, which is found in the skin of red grapes and therefore in many red wines, but the amount present is very small and that is why the supplements are extracted from Japanese Knotweed, a plant looking like bamboo and growing to be an invasive species.

Applied to yeast, worms, mice and fish, an increase in longevity and better genetic expression were proven. The effect was more noticeable in older species and not very effective in young specimens.

Some scientists published their conclusions in Cell Biology, highlighting the metabolic benefits of resveratrol as a result of the direct influence on the expression of genes that affect longevity, but only in those animals that have the longevity gene SIRT1. Researchers discovered that this ingredient has other effects, influencing dozens of other proteins critical for essential metabolic functions. It is attributed effects in increasing testosterone, improving diabetes, anti-inflammatory action, tumor reduction, neuroprotective and cardiac effects. However, there are hardly any recent experiences that support all these effects in humans. Taking into account that wine contains a reasonable alcohol content, we should be cautious when recommending this drink on healthy grounds.

So our advice is simple: if you want resveratrol, eat the skin of black grapes and chew their seeds.

COLOSTRUM

Colostrum is a thick, yellowish fluid of high density and low volume, secreted by the mammary glands during pregnancy, until the postpartum period. In these first days, a volume of 2-20 ml is produced per feeding, sufficient to meet the needs of the newborn. Colostrum has less energy, lactose, lipids, glucose, urea, water-soluble vitamins, PTH and nucleotides than breast milk. However, it contains more protein, sialic acid, fat-soluble vitamins E, A, K and carotenes. The content of minerals such as sodium, zinc, iron, sulfur, selenium, manganese and potassium is also higher in colostrum, and the calcium and phosphorus content varies depending on the mother and her diet. The concentration of free amino acids varies between colostrum, transition milk and milk.

Colostrum has a very high content of immunoglobulins, especially IgA, lactoferrin, cells (lymphocytes and macrophages), oligosaccharides, cytokines and other defensive factors. In this sense, it is worth highlighting the presence of Transfer Factors, molecules capable of transferring cellular immunity from immune individuals to non-immune individuals.

Each of the growth factors in colostrum helps stimulate cell and tissue growth by activating DNA formation. Unlike other supplements that provide only individual growth factors, colostrums combine a complete package of growth factors that work together synergistically.

Most of the anti-aging effects of GH hormone therapy are a result of increasing the body's concentration of IGF1 and IGF2, the most active ingredients found in colostrum. They also control how cells should grow and repair themselves.

MYOSTATIN INHIBITORS

Myostatin is a protein that consists of 375 amino acids in its molecular structure. It is present in vertebrates and is produced essentially in skeletal muscle, and is also known as growth differentiation factor 8. It is a member of the TGF-beta family. (Transforming Growth Factor)- designated transduction proteins that regulate cell growth, proliferation and differentiation.

This peptide that affects muscle growth, in previous research its inhibition has been caused through the use of pharmacological agents, being related to beneficial effects on muscle growth and strength.

Now the need arises to carry out an investigation of the functioning of this molecule in centenarians, with the aim of analyzing to what degree it affects the extreme longevity that a human being may or may not have.

In this sense, the frequency of this effect has been statistically higher in the centenarian population compared to the control group (7.1% versus 2.7% respectively for the study carried out in Spain and 7.6% versus 3 % for the study carried out in Italy). This leads us to determine that although lifestyle and environmental factors have a fundamental effect on the aging pattern, the myostatin polymorphism may play a key role in exceptional human longevity.

The results extracted from this research (according to the European University) have revealed the great power of epigenetics in determining our lives and lays the foundations for great scientific development in terms of genetics.

Myostatin inhibitors may be able to reverse muscle loss and decrease fibrosis, as well as the buildup of connective tissue in muscle that affects people with muscular dystrophy and can be a problem in aging and inactivity.

SULFORAPHANES

Currently, the attention of nutrition specialists is focused on compounds called glucosinolates, precursors of biomolecules such as sulforaphane (1-isothiocyanato-4-(methylsulfinyl)-butane), present in some cruciferous vegetables.

In reality, it is a phytochemical under study due to its antimicrobial, anticarcinogenic and chemopreventive properties, demonstrated in experimental animals. These properties are studied in relation to pathologies such as certain types of cancer or Parkinson's disease. For example, it reduces the number of cells in acute lymphoblastic leukemia in tests carried out "in vitro", according to research published in the journal "Plos One" by scientists from the Baylor College of Medicine (United States). It is also known that it increases the protective cells of the immune system called intraepithelial lymphocytes that are present in the stomach and skin, being the first protective barrier capable of protecting us from numerous infections.

Now, the best of all is that we are talking about a compound present in vegetables that we can include in our diet. Indeed, a characteristic of cruciferous plants is the synthesis of compounds rich in sulfur, such as glucosinolates. Glucosinolates are synthesized and stored in plants as relatively stable precursors of isothiocyanates.

The plants of the order Brassicales and the family Cruciferae or Brassicaceae, comprise around 350 genera and more than 2000 species, including some plants of culinary interest such as cabbage, collard greens, cabbage, cauliflower, Brussels sprouts and broccoli. Other crops in this family are radishes, wild mustard and numerous garden herbs, which are used to prepare condiments or garnishes, but their contribution of nutrients to the diet is minimal. For all these reasons, the National Cancer Institute of the United States has ranked broccoli first on the list of vegetables with general anti-cancer properties.

You have to eat broccoli, but there are two drawbacks, on the one hand, raw broccoli contains approximately 2000 mcg. of sulforaphane for each dose. After cooking, there are 600 mcg left. of sulforaphane, which represents a destruction of 70%. On the other hand, the plant loses its properties with conservation.

CYCLOASTRAGENOL

CA-98's (CAG) is an astragaloside IV aglycone that was first identified by examining extracts of Astragalus gallinaceus as a plant with anti-aging properties. The present study demonstrates that CAG stimulates telomerase activity and cell proliferation in human neonatal keratinocytes. The distinctive telomerase activation property of CAG led to the evaluation of its possible application in the treatment of neurological disorders, with good results.

CAG treatment not only induced the expression of bcl2, a CREB-regulated gene, but also the expression of telomerase reverse transcriptase in primary cortical neurons. Interestingly, oral administration of CAG for 7 days attenuated depressive-like behavior in experimental mice.

In conclusion, CAG stimulates telomerase activity in human neonatal keratinocytes and rat neuronal cells, and induces the activation of elements to combat the root aging problem and is believed to have a large number of beneficial health effects. It can slow down the degenerative processes related to aging, and this action alone can produce important positive health results.

Studies with twenty subjects revealed that the anti-aging physiological effects act quickly and effectively, thus reducing the visible signs of aging.

With the help of CA-98 cycloastragenol (CA), telomerase activity is activated, which helps human cells live longer and cell loss is reduced. Therefore, these enzymes play an important role, keeping cells younger for longer.

VITAMIN E (Alpha tocopherol)

This molecule is better known as vitamin E although it is made up of 7 other forms. Alpha tocopherol restores telomerase activity, protecting the integrity of telomeres, which could explain why vitamin E helps prevent heart disease and prostate cancer.

Vitamin E comes in 8 different forms, 4 tocopherols and 4 tocotrienols and the Tocotrienol Range.

These compounds act:

Reducing cholesterol oxidation

Maintaining healthy triglyceride levels

Helping to maintain normal blood pressure levels.

In one study, it was shown that telomeres increased in length by 16% after exposure to tocopherols.

LUTEIN AND ZEAXANTHIN

In a study published this year by the Austrian Society for Heart Attack Prevention that included 786 individuals, with a mean age of 66 years, it was shown that elevated blood concentrations of 3 of the 14 antioxidants tested: Lutein, Zeaxanthin and Vitamin C were associated with significantly with increased telomere length.

The researchers concluded that high concentrations of any of these 3 antioxidants in plasma are associated with an increase in telomere length in healthy, elderly people.

L-CARNITINE

This amino acid is stored mainly in the muscles and brain. Little of it is found in other organs and its concentration in the blood is low.

The body uses it to repair tissue damage and eliminate toxins. A Chinese study showed that its addition to fibroblasts in culture protects telomeres by reducing their shortening and extends the life cycle of the cells.

It also acts as a brain stimulant, increasing the level of neuronal growth factor up to 100 times more.

Elderly people show a marked reduction due to the body's limited synthesis capacity.

Acetyl L-Carnitine is used selectively to prevent brain aging.

L-ARGININE

The amino acid L-Arginine is recognized for improving blood flow. This is because it increases nitric oxide production and telomerase activity on the layer of epithelial cells that are housed on the inner walls of blood vessels.

The increase in telomerase activity, in turn, stimulates the production of nitric oxide. The expansion of these vessels and the increase in blood and oxygen that occurs is essential for life and sexual function in men.

N-ACETYL CYSTEINE

This amino acid is the basis for the organic synthesis of the main antioxidant, Glutathione. Additionally, N-Acetyl-Cysteine promotes telomerase activity and protects the integrity of telomeres, thus extending the lifespan of cells.

NAD

According to a new study, published in the journal "Science", a metabolite called 'nicotinamide adenine dinucleotide' (NAD+), which is found in all cells in the body, plays a key role in regulating protein interactions that control repair of the DNA damaged by radiation exposure or aging.

As David Sinclair, director of this research published in the journal "Science," explains, "the cells of the oldest mice were indistinguishable from those of the young animals after a single week of treatment." As David Sinclair highlights, "this is the closest we have come to an effective and safe anti-aging drug that, perhaps, will be on the market within three to five years if the clinical trial goes as it should."

INDOL-3-CARBINOL

Its properties on telomeres lie essentially in indole-3-carbinol, with a marked antiestrogenic effect and the possibility of inducing apoptosis in malignant cells. It corrects autoimmune diseases and it is believed that I-3-C can mimic the effects of calorie restriction and prolong lifespan by correcting damaged DNA.

Laboratory studies carried out to date indicate that this product blocks telomere shortening. On the other hand, in experiments it has been observed that I-3-C can cause the death of prostate cancer cells, without affecting healthy ones.

Indole-3-carbinol may also act as an anti-aging supplement, reducing damage caused by free radicals and supporting healthy cellular function. It may also reduce the risk of heart disease by preventing increased platelet aggregability and reducing the secretion of apolipoprotein B.

LIFESTYLE

Exercise

While nutritious eating represents an important link in a healthy lifestyle, exercise cannot be ignored, as there is evidence to suggest that it protects against telomere shortening. However, strenuous exercise, which is done without listening to the body's signals that invite us to rest, causes oxidative stress that increases aging. Although the muscles seem to respond to intense movement, the rest of the body suffers sometimes irreversible deterioration.

High-intensity exercise seems to be the favorite of many people, because their physical appearance makes them appear healthy, but little by little, the passing of the years leads to premature aging.

Hypocaloric diet

Previous research has shown that we can extend life by reducing calorie consumption, no more than 1,800/2,000. The problem is that the figures that appear in dietetics manuals and studies continue to speak of between 2,500 and 3,500, figures that could have been valid in the 40s and 50s, when the world population worked intensively more than 10 hours a day, not She had hardly any free days, she was raising numerous children, and the housing and clothing were inadequate.

Research conducted with laboratory rats has shown that simply decreasing carbohydrates and increasing protein activates the genes that govern youth and longevity.

Also, we can have similar health benefits in terms of calorie restriction, through intermittent fasting.

About the attack on alternative medicines.

Don't worry, my friends, because alternative medicines to chemicals will still be there, curing millions of people around the world.

Only an ignorant person can reject and mock the immense work of nature, and only an egomaniacal scientist dares to assure that he and his clumsy students can improve the process of creation.

Let's let everyone heal how and with whom they want, and keep in mind that, unless they destroy all the medicinal plants in the world and take away all the organic foods from us, we will continue to heal with them.

Adolfo Pérez Agustí

The author

OTHER BOOKS OF YOUR INTEREST

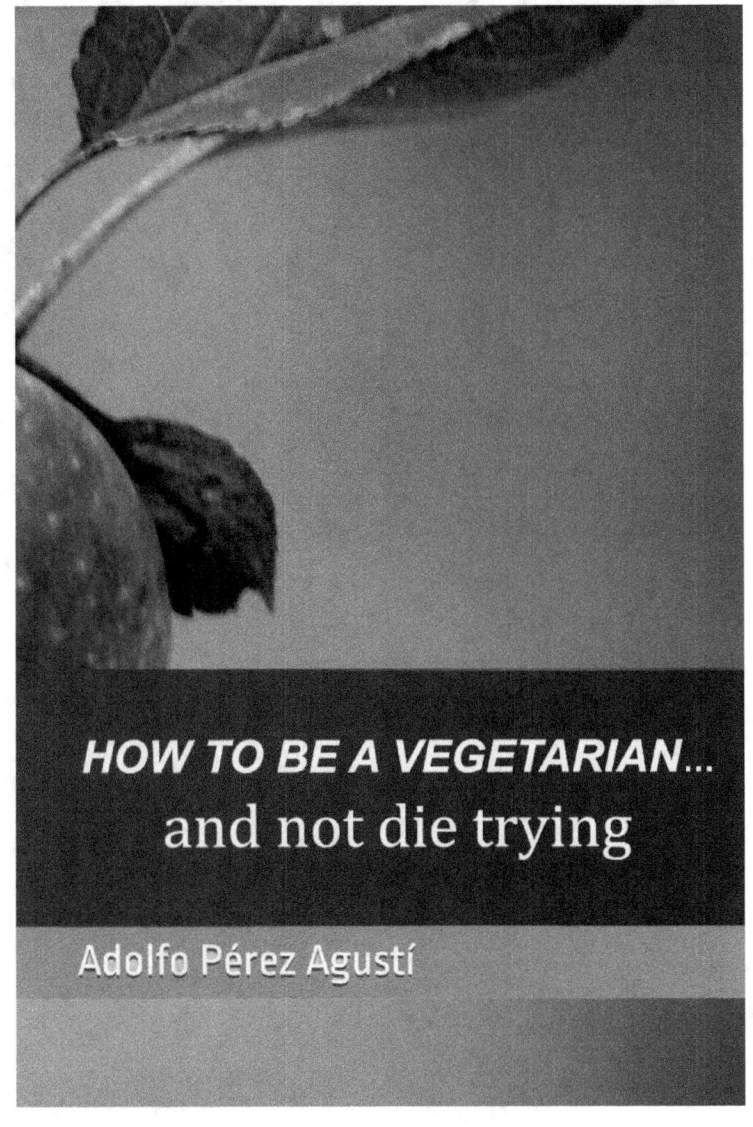

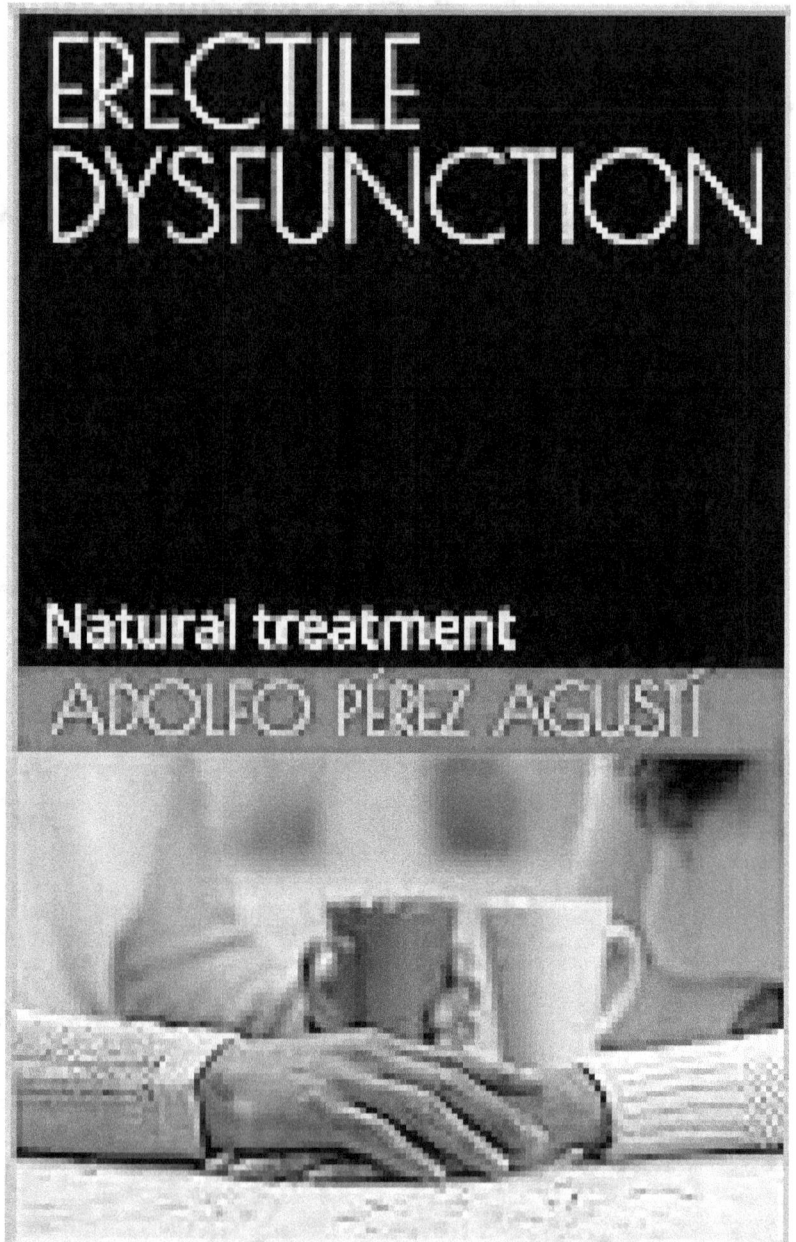

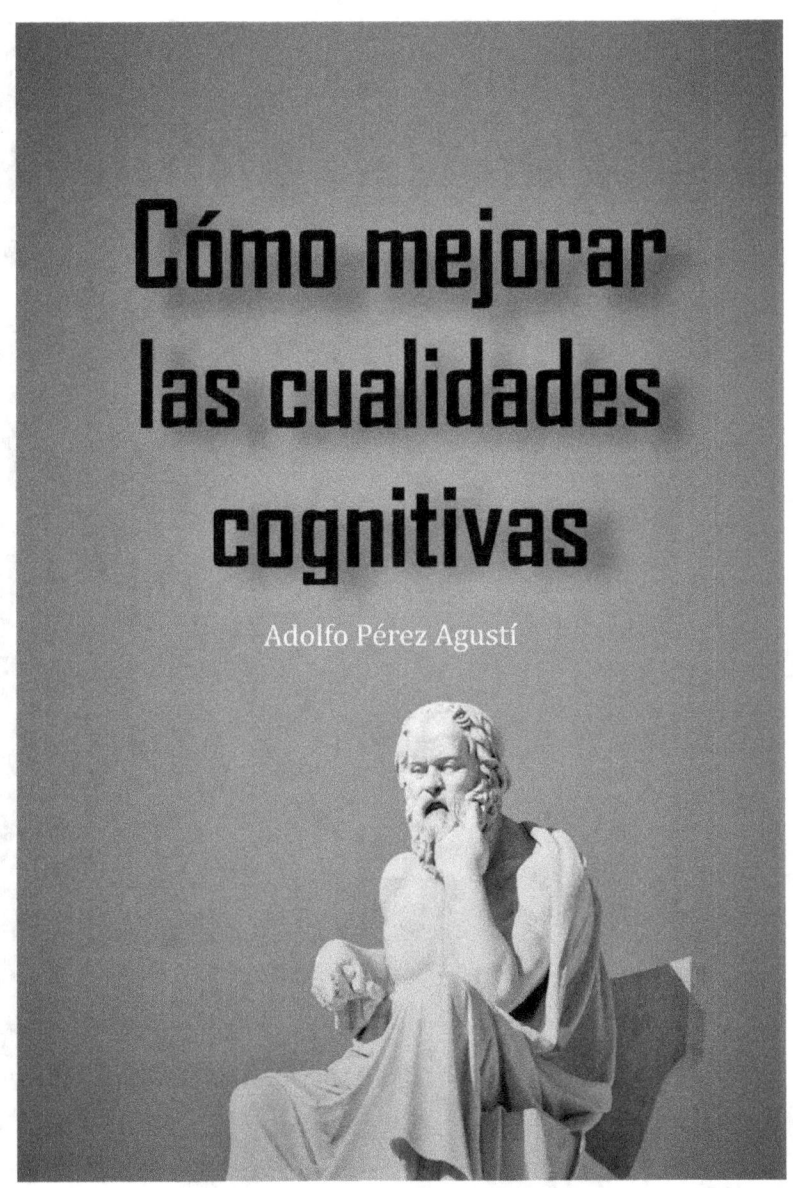

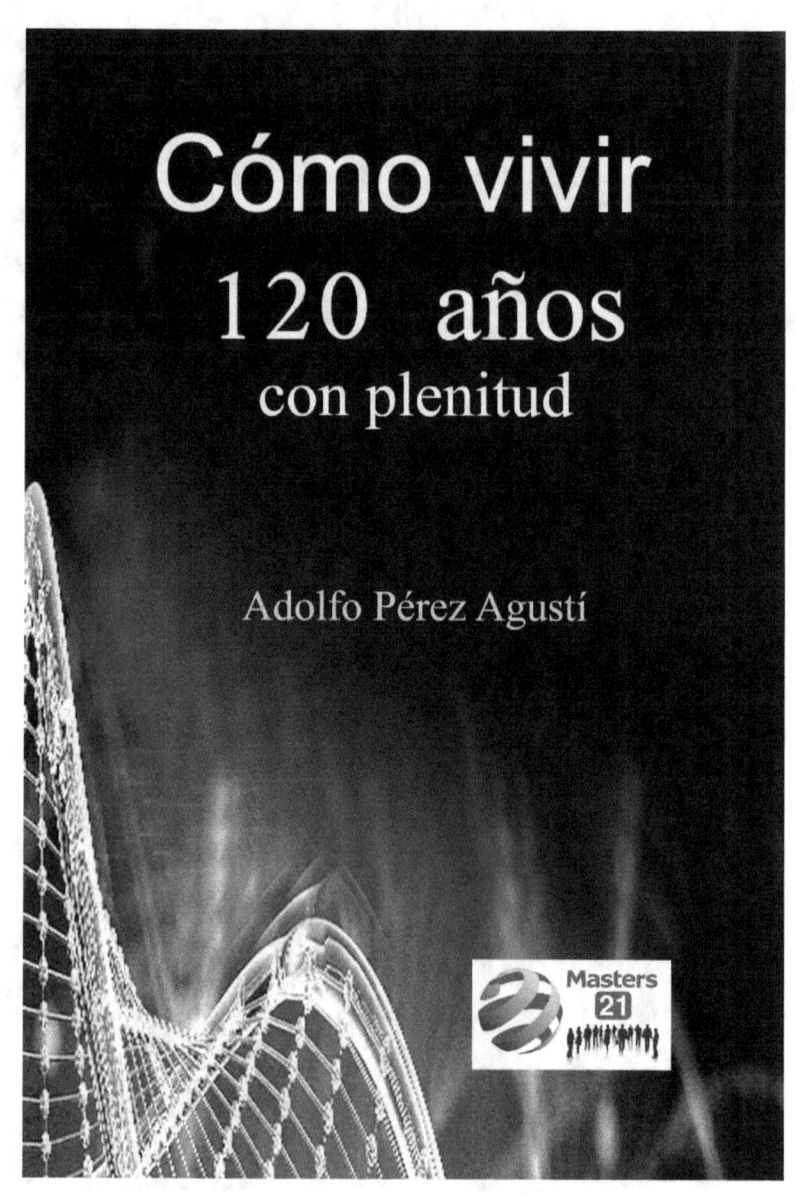

www.ingramcontent.com/pod-product-compliance
Lightning Source LLC
Chambersburg PA
CBHW052246220526
45471CB00001B/211